NUTRITION AND FOOD

Nutrition and Food

Udai Veer

ANMOL PUBLICATIONS PVT. LTD.
NEW DELHI - 110 002 (INDIA)

ANMOL PUBLICATIONS PVT. LTD.
4374/4B, Ansari Road, Daryaganj
New Delhi - 110 002
Ph.: 23261597, 23278000
Visit us at: www.anmolpublications.com

Nutrition and Food

First Published, 2005

ISBN 81-261-2486-5

PRINTED IN INDIA

Published by J.L. Kumar for Anmol Publications Pvt. Ltd., New Delhi - 110 002 and Printed at Mehra Offset Press, Delhi.

Contents

Preface

Nutrition is the basis of life and nutrition comes from food. Food preparation, food preservation and service of food, are all vital parts of modern day hotel industry.

The book titled : Nutrition and Food is a new and valuable addition to a handful of authentic books on the subject of Food Science. Being a research-based, exhaustive and comprehensive work, this book is bound to prove to be a good stuff for students, teachers, professionals and general readers.

Hopefully, this series of books would be acknowledged and accepted by the concerned circles. And that will really be a reward for the undersigned. He is confident of being admired for his endeavour.

Editor

1

Diet Plan

Everyone knows that good diet is needed to sustain good health. By health we mean the well-being of an individual in physical, emotional and social conditions. Just the presence or absence of a disease cannot label a person as healthy. Sound emotional and mental condition of an individual is contributed by good nutrition. A healthy person will have a positive attitude towards life. A good natured person full of life reflects his better health standards. A good or adequate diet is known as 'balanced diet'. A balanced diet yields daily nutrients in the proper amounts and proportion required by the body.

Nutritional Needs

Nutritional requirements vary according to age, sex, physical activities and other physiological conditions. The National Institute of Nutrition is engaged in research work on the dietary pattern of Indians and their requirements of various nutrients. The Nutrition Advisory Committee of the Indian Council of Medical Research made recommendations in 1944 for all nutrients. They were revised in 1958 and 1968. In 1980 further recommendations were made by the Nutrition Advisory Committee and the latest requirements are available now for formulating balanced diets for various groups. A balanced diet must supply enough food to the body for deriving energy. Energy is simply expressed as the capacity to do work. For basic activities like heart beat, breathing and excretion energy is required. Energy is stored as carbohydrate in foods. Cereals like rice, wheat, millets like ragi or bajra contain much carbohydrates in the form of starch. Starchyuits like banana and roots like tapioca, potato, yam, colocasia and sweet potato are rich in carbohydrates. Energy requirements for various age groups are given elsewhere and for an adult sedentary man 2,400 kcals are required and for a sedentary woman 1,900 kcals are recommended. In a balanced diet energy from cereals should not exceed more than 75 per cent of total requirements. Energy derived from fat or oil should not exceed 15 per cent of the total calories and from refined carbohydrates (sugar and jaggery) has been recommended around 5 per cent of the total calories.

A balanced diet must supply enough protein for building up our tissues in various parts of our body. When some tissurs get worn out or used up proteins repair and replace them. Proteins are essential for the secretion of digestive juices and synthesis of enzymes and hormone production. Dietary proteins are used again for the synthesis of body ins. Protein requirements must be met by dietary proteins. Usually in requirement is in terms of body weight, that is, 1 gm of protein to body weight is the recommendation. Even though animal ins are of superior quality it is not a practical suggestion to depend on them for dietary proteins. In an average Indian diet pulses are a very important source of proteins. When nutritional scores are given to jus proteins egg has a high score of 90 per cent whereas vegetable proteins score only 45 to 50 per cent in the case of pulses and 45 per cent to cereals. But it can be improved by incorporating pulse and cereal proteins; 40 to 60 gms of pulses and 150 to 250 ml of milk can provide enough proteins in a vegetarian diet For non-vegetarians 20 to 30 gms of pulses and one egg or 30 gms of meat or fish and 100 to 150 ml of k provide the protein requirement If no pulse is used non-elarians can take two eggs or 50 gms of meat or fish or 30 gms of fish neat and one egg.

Fats and oils are other major nutrients in a balanced diet. Fats are icentrated forms of energy. Fat soluble vitamins are utilised only in presence of fat For males 40 to 65 gms of fat and for females 20 to gms of fat must be included in a balanced diet. Vitamins are essential the proper functioning of our body. Small quantities of vitamins own dramatic effect on our body. Organs like eyes, alimentary canal, in and mucous membraneous structures depend on vitamins for their formal structure and functions. Leafy vegetables, other vegetables, yellow vegetables and roots and tubers provide almost all the vitamins required by our body. About a quarter kilogram of vegetables is required in our daily diet to ensure vitamin supply. Raw vegetables or sprouted grams or fruits are essential to supply vitamin C. Minerals like calcium, phosphorus, iron and trace elements and salts are essential to maintain good health. Sodium chloride is essential to regulate water metabolism in our body. A balanced diet provides enough vitamins and minerals from natural sources. Tonics or supplements are not required or people who consume balanced diets. The Indian Council of Medical Research has designed Recommended Dietary Allowances for various nutrients. They have also formulated composition of balanced diet for various groups. These allowances are designed to serve as a guideline for planning diets. Suggestions are given for substituting foods for-non-vegetarians and additional allowances during special conditions.

To include the above nutrients in daily diet certain guidelines are suggested by the ICMR. Food items which contribute the same nutrients are grouped together and certain food groups are evolved. Foods are grouped into 11 groups based on their nutritive value. They are cereals and millets, pulses, nuts and oilseeds, vegetables, fruits, milk and milk products, meat, fish, eggs and poultry, fats and oils, sugar and jaggery and spices and condiments.

Cereals and millets constitute 70 to 80 per cent of calories and proteins of low income group. Except ragi all cereals are poor in calcium. Dried pulses are rich in proteins and a cereal-pulse combination is an excellent substitute for animal proteins—pulses are also good sources of many B vitamins and sprouting enhances the vitamin C content of pulses. Nuts and oilseeds are good sources of proteins, certain B vitamins, vitamin E and minerals like phosphorus andiron.

Vegetables are the storehouse of carotene, riboflavin, folic acid, vitamin C and calcium. Vegetables also supply water and roughage to the body. Leafy vegetables, other vegetables and roots and tubers are the different types of vegetables. Fruits in general are a good source of vitamin C. Milk is nature's best food as it is almost complete except for iron and vitamin 'C. Like milk, egg also contains proteins of high biological value. Egg is a rich source of vitamin A and some B vitamins. Animal foods like meat, fish and poultry are rich sources of proteins and B vitamins. Fatty fish are good in fat, vitamin A and D and small fish with bones are good sources of calcium. Liver and other organ meats are good sources of proteins, vitamin A, B complex, B12 and iron.

Sugar and jaggery are good sources of energy and honey and jaggery contain minerals like iron. Condiments and spices are mainly used to enhance palatability.

For non-vegetarians pulses can be reduced to 50 per cent and instead of that, one egg or 30 gms of meat or fish can be included. If no pulse is taken two eggs or 50 gms of meat or fish can be included.

Ideal Diet

For planning a balanced diet for labourers, low cost nutritious foods must be included. Ragi, tapioca, sweet potato, clusterbeans, bittergourd, soyabeans, drumstick leaves, various types of leafy vegetables, cowgram, horsegram, groundnut, Indian gooseberry, guava, papaya, mango, cashew fruit and other seasonal fruits can be used liberally to make a low-cost balanced diet Sprouted pulses and cheap vegetables that can be used as raw salads also must be included to meet the vitamin C requirement.

The ICMR Advisory Committee (1981) recommended the composition of balanced diet and it is given below:

Food Item	*Adult Man*			*Adult Woman*		
	Seden-tary	*Moderate Work*	*Heavy Work*	*Seden-tary*	*Moderate Work*	*Heavy Work*
Cereals	460 gm	520 gm	670 gm	410 gm	440 gm	575 gm
Pulses	40 gm	50 gm	60 gm	40 gm	45 gm	50 gm
leafy vegetables	40 gm	40 gm	40 gm	100 gm	100 gm	100 gm

Contd...

Food Item	*Adult Man*			*Adult Woman*		
	Seden-tary	*Moderate Work*	*Heavy Work*	*Seden-tary*	*Moderate Work*	*Heavy Work*
Other vegetables	60 gm	70 gm	80Lgrn	40 gm	40 gm	100 gm
Roots and tubers	50 gm	60 gm	80 gm	50 gm	50 gm	100 gm
Milk and milk products	150 ml	200 ml	250 ml	100 ml	150 ml	200 ml
Oil and fat	40 gm	45 gm	65 gm	20 gm	25gm	40 gm
Fruits	60 gm	60 gm	60 gm	60 gm	60 gm	60 gm
Sugar and jaggery	30 gm	35 gm	55 gm	20 gm	20 gm	40 gm

For non-vegetarians pulses 5O per cent less + one egg or 30 gms fish or meat, if no pulse, 2 eggs or 50 gm fish or meat.

A Sample Diet for a Sedentary Woman

Time		*Meal*		*Menu*
6.30 a.m.	-	Bed coffee		
8 a.m.	-	Breakfast	-	Chapathi, Groundnuts-Tomato curry, Coffee
12.30 Noon	-	Lunch	-	Rice or Chapathi, Brinjal and horsegram curry Amaranth or spinach pugath, Lassi, Carrot salad.
4 p.m.	-	Tea	-	Vegetable vermicelli uppuma, Mint leaf chutney, Tea.
8 p.m.	-	Dinner	-	Wheat dosa or phulkas, Sprouted green gram curry, Fruit cup.

Quantities of various food groups can be distributed according to the composition given by ICMR. This above diet provides:

Calories - 2420kcals

Proteins - 53 gms

The idea that the body's needs are definite and can be measured is a very recent one. We are so accustomed to eating to satisfy hunger that for centuries this criterion accepted by most people without question. Plenty was, in general, associated with health and want with starvation.

And yet, throughout the ages there have been those few who have seen a little further into the meaning of nutrition. We know from the book of Daniel of how he asked that he and his companions might eat a simple diet of pulses and water and how, after ten days during which this was permitted, 'their countenances appeared fairer and fatter in flesh than all the children which did eat the portion of the king's meat.' This was probably the first dietary experiment ever to be recorded.

We also know how, in the Middle Ages, illness and loss of life from scurvy led to the recognition that food could prevent and cure certain diseases but the connection between man's daily food and his health was only dimly acknowledged and in a very limited field.

Fortunately, the pleasures of a mixed diet led those who could afford it to eat a variety of foods. The greater the variety, the greater chance there was that all the vital and necessary factors would be included. Hence disease was most prevalent in institutions where the food was restricted and monotonous and among the poor who could not afford variety.

It was Sanctorius (1561-1636) who showed, by sitting on a chair suspended from the arm of a balance while he ate a meal, that afterwards the increase in weight which had taken place was gradually lost again. He described the loss as due to 'insensible perspiration.'

This proved the first basic fact that body-weight was connected with food eaten and that living, even without any conscious exertion, causes loss of weight.

This led in time to the acknowledgment that all the activities of the body derived their energy from the slow combustion of the foods eaten or (in starvation) of the body itself.

An adequate diet is one of that provides all the essential nutrients in sufficient quantities to meet the needs of the body. Thus far, the energy and nutrient needs, including carbohydrates, fats, proteins, minerals, vitamins, and water. The information concerning each of the nutrients in terms of the day's food is now brought together. Easy rule-of-thumb methods for knowing which foods and how much of each one are needed to provide an adequate diet have been developed on the basis of *food groups;* for this purpose, foods similar in nutritive value are considered together as a group. The pattern for the adequate diet is developed by recommending sufficient food servings from the various groups.

Human Requirements

The food shortages during and after the 1914-18 war and the resulting ill-health of children, especially in Eastern Europe, made the general public realize for the first time that starvation was not the only consequence of a poor diet. Enough food to satisfy hunger sometimes failed to protect from diseases of malnutrition. Food had to be of the right and, to be fully protective, had to contain the essential vitamins as well as the basic nutrients : proteins, fats, carbohydrates and mineral salts.

Information to have extracted from old records about diets known to have been associated with deficiency diseases. Beriberi had occurred most commonly in countries where rice formed the bulk of the food eaten and had been known to disappear when some of the rice was replaced by vegetables. A diet provided for the U.S.A. garrison of Porto Rico consisted of rice, beans, potatoes, onions and meat with some extra fruit and vegetables, and on this, cases of beriberi occurred. Using recent values for the vitamins B_1 content of these foods, we find that the daily diet contained about 0.5 mg. of vitamin B_1 per man.

This represents an average intake, and implies the some men ate less and some more, the former being without doubt those who succumbed to beriberi. The rations were later improved. Less rice and onions were given and more beans, potatoes and meat, and with the change, beriberi disappeared from the camp. The vitamin B_1 of the improved ration calculated by modern methods was just over 0.8 mg. per man — an increase of only 0.3 mg. but it made the difference between beriberi and protection. This difference is about two-millions of the total weight of a man's daily food, so it is not surprising that vitamins, active in such minute amounts, remained undiscovered for so long.

During the 19th century, scurvy was common in prisons and in other institutions, not to be punitive. In 1822 the meals in Millbank Penitentiary are described as:

For females — morning 9 oz. bread
¾ pint gruel (made with barley)
noon 9 oz. bread ¾ pint soup evening ¾ pint soup.

The bread would have been made from stone-ground flour and would contain plenty of vitamin B_1, so as we should expect, there is a history of beriberi in such a prison, but any vegetables used in the preparation of the soup would be unlikely to retain any vitamin C during the cooking and it recorded that 448 prisoners did in fact show signs of scurvy in one year.

During the war of 1914-18, both scurvy and beriberi occurred. Soldiers of the Indian Army who ate few vegetables and little if any meat, suffered from scurvy. The British on the other hand, who ate vegetables, but while in India had rice or refined cereals, went down with beriberi. In 1916, special hospitals for the admission of cases of scurvy were operated in Baghdad and other parts of the Middle East.

A valuable study was made between 1920 and 1930 on the effect of increasing the quantities of protective foods in the meals of schoolboys. Records were kept of the heights and weights of boys between the ages of 10 and 18 at a large public school. Conditions of housing, the amount of physical exercise taken and other possibly influential factors remained relatively constant during period and the boys were, by accepted standards of nutrition, well fed. However as a result of an increasing awareness of the importance of vitamin-containing food the authorities altered the diet, so that the boys ate less bread and more milk, vegetables and butter. The results of these changes as seen in records kept over a long period were published by the medical officer (Friend, 1935).

At all ages there was an increase in both height and weight, this being greatest, as one would expect, during the years of most rapid growth.

It may be argued that increase in size does not necessarily mean better health and we are all familiar with overweight children who are abnormally fat but, in general, and where large numbers are concerned, the rate of growth of children can be taken as one indication of physical progress.

This study as important a being the first of its kind undertaken on an adequate scale and over a long enough period to give reliable results.

With the increasing consumption of vegetables and fruits in Great Britain, scurvy, at one time described as the 'English disease,' became rare and the introduction of cod liver oil as a supplement for infants reduced the incidence of rickets, but the new knowledge of the importance of vitamins as protective factors roused great interest in nutrition and people began to wonder how present-day diets would stand up tests of adequacy.

The first report of a large-scale investigation into modern diets was published by J. Boyd Orr in 1937. He divided the community into six sections according to income and estimated the amounts of money spent on food and also the consumption of protective foods in the different income groups. He found that with rise of income, more protective foods were eaten and that in three lowest groups, the amounts of Vitamins A and C eaten were very low.

Investigations on similar lines were made in the United States and from all the data collected, it became possible to make a fairly good estimate of the amounts of the more common vitamins contained in the daily food of normal healthy people and also the amounts below which deficiency diseases were liable to occur.

Tables setting out probable human requirements were published by a Technical Commission of the League of Nations in 1937 and by the Government Bureau of Home Economics, U.S.A. (Stiebeling, 1933). This was before the adoption in the United States of international units, so the results are not comparable but the attempt to express human needs in terms of quantities of vitamins was in itself a great advance.

Later, tables using international units were prepared by the National Research Council of the U.S.A. and these gave (except for vitamin C) figures surprisingly close to the League of Nations recommendations. The most recent publication is that the British Medical Association, 1950.

	League of Nations 1937	*National Research Council 1945*	*British Medical Assoc, 1950*
Vitamin A	2,000-4,000 i.u.	5,000 (optimum)	i.u. 3,000 i.u.
Vitamin B_1	1 mg. approx.	1.5 mg.	1.4 mg.
Vitamin C	30 mg	75 mg.	20 mg.
Vitamin D	—	—	400 i.u.

During the war of 1939-45 there were many cases of dietary deficiency including beriberi in the Japanese prison camps. Some of the doctors who were among the prisoners kept record of the occurrence of beriberi and also of the vitamin B_1 of the diet and the history of the Porto Rico garrison was repeated. When the intake fell blow 0.5 mg. vitamin B_1 (or about 0.2 mg. per 1,000 nonfat Calories) men succumbed to beriberi; when it rose above these levels, the men's health improved (Smith and others, 1951).

The Register-General's Statistical Review which is published every year gives details of the number of deaths from different diseases. Although the causes of scurvy and rickets were known in the 1920s, and the foods effective for prevention were available, the diseases did not disappear immediately. There was, however, a steady drop in incidence. This demonstrates that not only must protective foods be available, but the public must be educated to use them properly. Free supplements for the provision of vitamins A, C and D were made available for infants during the war years but all mothers did not avail themselves of the opportunity to have them. The number taking them has increased considerably in the last few years with a corresponding drop in rickets almost to the point of disappearance (Registrar-General, 1949, 1950 and 1952) and the health of children in this country has steadily improved.

Health and Illnesses

Most of the vitamins, being growth-promoting substances in the sense that they are needed for full structural and functional development are needed greater amounts during childhood when growth is taking place and during pregnancy and lactation for the same reason.

Vitamin A : Vitamin A is stored in the liver and during adult life the daily needs can be supplied to a considerable extent from these reserves. Volunteers who deliberately consumed diets very low in vitamin A were able to continue doing so for several months without developing any gross signs of deficiency. But in spite of this there is general agreement that it is better to consume enough to guard against any chances of deficiency and, in the table, the recommended levels of vitamin A vary very little.

Whether taken as vitamin A itself or in the plant form carotene, this factor is always converted into vitamin A used as such in the animal body. But the two forms are not of equal physiological value, unit for unit. It is usually reckoned that the number of international units needed in the form of carotene is about twice the number needed as vitamin A itself. Even this ratio is not the same for all foods. The carotene of green vegetables supplies to the body about half as many units of vitamin A as the number obtained by chemical estimation, but yellow vegetables like carrots supply only about one-fifth or one-quarter (Graves, 1942).

Increased Needs for the Vitamin A : Vitamin A being used by the body to maintain the health of the skin, teeth and mucous linings of the respiratory organs is needed especially in illness in which these are involved. To guard against them, supplies in the daily diet should be kept up to the standards given. In treatment higher doses are available in pharmaceutical preparations can be prescribed. Dases up to 100,000 or 200,000 i.u. are sometimes given daily.

The B Vitamins : The need for vitamin B_1 varies according to the amount of food eaten and the energy expended in movements in all kinds.

As muscular activity, which depends on the oxidation of carbohydrates, continues throughout life, vitamin B_1 must be continuously supplied. Moreover, this vitamin differs from vitamin A is not being stored for long periods. In general, the fat-soluble vitamins tend to be stored in the body, but the water-soluble vitamins, i.e. those of the B group and vitamin C, are not stored. If more is eaten than needed it is rapidly excreted again in the urine.

Because vitamin B_1 is used day by day, as it is consumed, it has been much easier to find out exactly what the daily needs are in fact, as early as 1934, Cowgill was able to suggest a mathematical formula to express the daily needs in terms of body weight and calorific intake.

Increased Needs for Vitamin B : As vitamin B_1 is concerned with carbohydrate metabolism, any conditions which involve a higher calorific intake, e.g heavy manual work, climbing, Article exploration, naturally call for higher intake.

In those diseases, too, in which the rate of metabolism is increased, more vitamin B_1 is needed.

Riboflavin and nicotinic acid also take part with vitamin B_1 in energy relations and the amounts needed are related to the amount of vitamin B_1 In foods, these vitamins of the B complex occur together and a shortage of one usually implies a shortage of the others. It is only when the staple cereal happens to be grossly short of a particular factor as, for example, polished rice and vitamin B_1 or maize and nicotinic acid, that well-defined deficiency diseases such as beriberi and pellagra occur. In countries where mixed diets are customary, deficiencies are usually less severe but of a mixed type. For example, a mild shortage of riboflavin will produce, in some individuals, roughness and redness of the skin over the nose and some cracking of the lips, easily cured by the consumption of extra quantities of one or two foods rich in riboflavin such as eggs or liver.

Similarly a shortage of nicotinic acid, not enough to cause pellagra, may produce digestive disturbances, a reddening of the skin of the face and hands and feelings of depression.

Nicotinic acid is concerned in healthy people with the control of movements of precision and if its supply is limited subjects may find themselves unusually clumsy.

The varying responses of individuals to diets deficient in the B vitamins was puzzling until, as a result of a long series of observations, it was learnt that these factors are also synthesized within the body of man and the higher animals though not by it. The intestinal tract contains warm semifluid material rich in nutrients and is, as we know, a medium in which there is normally an expensive bacterial flora. These organisms are not disease-producing. They merely live in and with man. Their power of synthesizing vitamins is a relatively recent discovery. They seem to specialize in the factors of the B group but some can also synthesize vitamin K (Najjar and Barrett, 1945).

Ruminants, whose large rumen in the first part of the digestive tract is the site of vitamin formation, obtain so much riboflavin and nicotinic acid from bacterial activity that they fail to develop rings of deficiency even on diets lacking these vitamins. But in man the bacteria carry on their synthetic activities much further down the digestive tract and, although undoubtedly some of the B vitamins produced in this way are available for human use, enough of each is not formed to satisfy all human needs.

It is, however easy to see that in conditions such as diarrhoea in which the contents of the alimentary tract move along quickly, less than the normal amounts may be absorbed and symptoms of deficiency may occur if the condition is not checked. The recent use of some of the new drugs, sulphonamides and antibiotics has also revealed that these, too, affect the activities of the vitamin-B-producing bacteria. The drugs inhibit not only the growth of disease-producing organisms but also the synthesis of the B vitamins in the intestine. This interference with production may be great enough to cause true secondary deficiencies in patients who may not have been very well supplied with vitamins before. Cases have been observed with signs of peripheral neuritis, enlarged heart and swelling of the limbs, indistinguishable from true beriberi. Other patients develop a sore mouth and red scaling of the skin recalling deficiencies of nicotinic acid and riboflavin.

In the treatment of these secondary deficiencies very large doses have to be given — a hundred or more times the amount needed for normal health.

Vitamin C : Vitamin C, also water-soluble, is another vitamin which should be taken daily, although the body stores are not exhausted as rapidly as those of vitamin B_1.

There is difference of opinion about the amount of vitamin C needed to maintain health. The American in which estimate is higher than the British. An experiment in which volunteers did without any vitamin C for months showed that they could do so without developing any gross signs of scurvy, and the quantity needed for health has consequently been placed at a lower level than formerly. But, as the signs of deficiency develop in such an insidious manner, it is probable that minor degrees of vitamin C deficiency are fairly common though not always recognized as such.

It is known now that vitamin C is concerned not only in protection against scurvy but in the healing of wounds, in the prevention of shock from injury, in the tolerance of high atmospheric temperature and in the control of body fluids. These processes are common in everyday life and probably account for the daily use by the body of vitamin C.

Increased Needs for Vitamin C : When any of these, conditions are actually present or exaggerated the need is correspondingly increased. Very large doses (up to 1 g.) are given before operation to prevent shock and in the treatment of severe injuries and larger than normal doses are given to man doing heavy work in an excessively hot humid atmosphere.

Large amounts of vitamin C are available in fruits and vegetables and some reason or other an individual does not eat or can not eat these foods, then tablets of the synthetic vitamin or some other pharmaceutical preparation must be taken. The massive doses are, of course, always given by means of a pharmaceutical preparation.

Vitamin D : It will be noticed that the table gives the same figure for the human requirement for vitamin D except in the case of infants under one year and for expectant and nursing mothers. This uniform level is an fact a confession that very little is known about varying needs.

At one time it was assumed that vitamin D was needed only

during the period of active growth. This view is no longer held and it is thought that the fragile nature of the bones people of older may be related to their low consumption of vitamin D foods.

The figures for human needs given in the B.M.A. table have been obtained by studies of dietary surveys, of individual diets, of diets associated with deficiency diseases and so on. The first estimates were made by the Health Committee of the League of Nations; these were followed by American estimates and finally the table quoted here was produced. Considering the magnitude and difficulty of the task, it is astonishing how closely the various estimates agree and it is probable that these recently published figures are as near the truth as we are likely to get.

The question has to be asked : to what extent do individuals eat diets which satisfy these needs? How easy or difficult is it to obtain an adequate diet?

There are several ways of approaching this problem. We can see whether there is any evidence that people are better fed now than formerly or we can study foods which are normally eaten in ordinary homes and see if they supply the needs.

Reference has been made to the effect of adding protective foods to the diet of schoolboys and to the increases in height and weight produced as a result. Data on the height and weights of London school children during the first half of this century have recently been published and these show the same kind of increase. It may not be totally due to nutrition, but it is not unreasonable to conclude that improved feeding due to increased knowledge of nutrition has also played a part in producing these effects.

If we approach the problem from the dietary angle, we can analyse representative diets and estimate their vitamin content. This is a useful exercise and a comparison between the foods eaten on several different days or by different individuals shows how wide the variation in vitamin content can be.

Following examples of meals will illustrate this point. These show that the value of a diet depends on the *choice* of foods, and that likes and dislikes are of themselves not reliable guides; there must be knowledge also.

Amount *Oz.*		*Vit. A or equiv. in carotene* *i.u.*	*Vit.* B_1 *µg.*	*Ribo flavin* *µg.*	*Niacin* *µg.*	*Vit C* *mg.*	*Vit D* *i.u.*
Meal 1							
Roast beef	3	42	33	195	3,900	—	
Yorkshire pudding							
3 oz. = flour	1	_	34	23	450	-	-
milk	1½	45	18	54	-	-	0.45
egg	½	125	19	85	-	-	8.5
cooking fat	1/8	-	-	-	-	-	-
Roast potatoes	6	-	180	26	1,200	15	-
Cabbage	4	288*	4	28	320	28	-
Apple pie= flour	½	-	17	11	225	-	
cooking fat	¼	-	-	-	-	-	
apple	2	4	6	-	50	1.6	-
sugar	¼	-	-	-	-	-	
Custard= milk	2	60	24	72	-	-	0.6
powder	neg	-	-	-	-	-	-
		564	335	564	6,145	44.6	9.55
		i.u.	µg.=	µg.=	µg.	= mg	i.u.
			.335	.564	6.145		
			mg.	mg.	mg.		
Proportion of day's need approx.		1/8	¼	1/3	½	All	1/40
Meal 2							
Cheese	1	369	9	140	100	-	4
Lettuce	2	727*	34	40	200	6	-
Tomato	3	540*	60	30	300	21	-
Wholemeal bread	3	-	270	150	1,800	-	-
Butter	½	568	-	-	-	-	8.5
Orange	3	48	60	30	300	48	-

Contd...

	Amount Oz.	Vit. A or equiv. in carotene i.u.	Vit. B_1 µg.	Ribo-flavin µg.	Niacin µg.	Vit C mg.	Vit D i.u.
Coffee= milk and sugar	5	150	60	180	-	1	1.5
		2,402 i.u.	493 µg.= .493 mg.	570 µg.= .57 mg.	2,700 µg.= 2.7 mg.	76 mg.	14 i .u.
Proportion of day's need approx		¾	1/3	1/3	1/5	All	1/90
Meal 3							
Fried white fish	4	-	40	160	2,400	-	-
Fried potatoes	6	-	180	60	1,200	12	-
Rice pudding 4 oz.							
= rice	1/3	-	5	6	100	-	-
milk	2½	75	30	90	-	-	.75
sugar	1/6	-	-	-	-	-	-
Stewed apple, 4 =raw	3	7	9	-	75	2.4	-
		82 i.u.	264 µg.= .264 mg.	316 µg.= .316 mg.	3,775 µg.= 3.775 mg.	14.4 mg.=	.75 i.u.
Proportion of day's need approx		1/40	1/5	1/6	1/4	1/2	negli-gible
Meal 4							
Sausages, pork	3	-	210	150	1,500	-	-
Baked beans	3	35	60	30	600	-	-
Mashed potatoes	6	-	144	96	1,350	12	-

Contd...

Amount *Oz.*	*Vit. A or equiv. in carotene* *i.u.*	*Vit. B_1* *µg.*	*Ribo-flavin* *µg.*	*Niacin* *µg.*	*Vit C* *mg.*	*Vit D* *i.u.*	
Prunes	4	103	32	68	-	-	-
Custard= milk powder	3	90	36	108	-	-	.9
		228 i.u.	482 µg.= .482 mg.	452 µg.= 4.52 mg.	3,450 µg. 3.45 mg.	12 = mg.	.9 i.u.
Proportion of day's need approx		1/13	1/3	1/4	1/4	3/5	negli-gible

For green vegetables : Carotene =40 per cent as vitamin A

Yellow veg. =25 per cent

Half the value of uncooked flour.

Where no value is available for vitamin B_1 in cooked food, the figure for the uncooked food is halved.

Units at Global Level

Vitamins A and D are usually expressed in international units (i.u.)- Human or animal requirements for other vitamins are usually given in milligrammes, but the value in foods is often expressed in microgrammes (1/1000s of miligramme) so as to avoid the use of decimals.

In the tables, the value of *individual* foods are given in microgrammes for the same reason but the *total* values and the requirements are given in milligrammes for comparison with other published figures.

Conversions —Weight and Household Measures

5 oz. milk	= 1 teacupful
1 oz. cheese is the same size as	1 oz. butter (1/4 of 1/4- 1b. pack)
1 oz. bread	= ¼ in. slice from square loaf

1 oz. cake	= portion 3 x 1 x 1 /2 in.
1 oz. Castle pudding is the same size as 1 oz. cake	
1 oz. biscuits	= 2 biscuits (2 1 /4 in. in diameter)
1 oz. flour, rice, oatmeal, custard, powder, sugar, etc.	= 1 well heaped tablespoonful
½ oz.	= 1 level tablespoonful or 1 well heaped teaspoonful
1 oz. jam	= 1 dessertspoonful
2 oz. potato (mashed), green vege. tables, root vegetables or peas	= 1 heaped tablespoonful
2 oz. tomato	= 1 egg-size tomato
4 oz. stewed fruit	= 5 small plumps (with juice) or 4 tablespoonfuls of soft fruit
3 oz. meat	= 4 thin slices (approx. 3 x 4 in.)
1 oz. bacon	= 1 rasher (approx. 1/8 x 7 x 2 in.)
4 oz. fish	= portion approx. 3 x 3 x 1/2 in.
2 oz. herring	= 1 small herring (approx.5 in. long)

2

Sufficient Diet

A plan for selecting an adequate diet developed around 4 *food groups* will now be discussed. There are other plans, developed on the same principle as the 4-group plan, differing only in number of groups. All of the plans are developed in accordance with food habits of the people and the foods available to them. In case the habits of eating and the food supply are different, the food patterns are of necessity also different.

The 4-group plan is flexible, permitting for a wide choice of foods within most of the groups. Meals planned in one home are likely to differ from those in another, even though the meals in each home follow the same food pattern. Foods selected by persons eating out may vary widely, and still at the same time each is in complete accordance with the recommendations of the same food pattern.

Four-food Group Plan : The 4-group plan (milk, meat, vegetable-fruit, cereal) was developed in 1958 and is a simplified version of the 7-group plan that originated during wartime 1943. In this 4-group plan the citrus fruits, green and yellow vegetables, and other vegetables and fruits are combined into one group, and the butter fortified margarine group omitted. The daily quantities of each group of recommended to provide the *foundation* of an adequate diet and the main nutritive contribution of each group are given.

Calories are the least well supplied by this pattern. However, as a usual practice, facts and sugars, which are not listed, are eaten as such or combined in baked goods and desserts, with a result that the energy intake is increased. Also to satisfy the appetite, additional servings from the food groups may be expected, which will contribute both to the energy and nutrient intake.

The 7 food groups	*Daily amounts*	*Min nutritive contributions*
Green and yellow vegetables	1 or more servings	Vitamin A value Ascorbic acid Iron
Oranges, grapefruit, tomatoes or raw cabbage or salad greens	1 serving	Ascorbic acid
Potatoes, other vegetables and fruits	2 or more servings	Vitamins and minerals in general Cellulose

The 7 food groups	*Daily amounts*	*Min nutritive contributions*
Milk and milk products	Children ¾ to 1 quart Adults 1 pint	Calcium Riboflavin Protein Phosphorus
Meat, poultry, fish and eggs	1 serving meat, fish or poultry 1 egg (at least 4 a week)	Protein Phosphorus Iron B- Vitamins
Bread, flour and cereal (whole grain enriched or restored)	3 or more servings	Thiamine Niacin Riboflavin Iron Carbohydrate Cellulose
Butter or fortified margarine	2-3 tbsp.	Vitamin A Fat

The basic 7 food groups.

Contd...

The 4 food groups contributions	*Daily amounts*	*Main nutritive*
Milk group:	Children 3-4 cups	
Milk, cheese, rice	Teen agers 4 or more cups	Calcium
cream (cheese and	Adults 2 or more cups	Riboflavin
ice cream can replace		
part of the milk)	Pregnant 4 or more cups	Protein
	Women	
	Nursing 6 or more cups	Phosphorus
	Mothers	
Meal group	Protein	
Beef veal pork, lamon,		Phosphorus
Poultry, fish, eggs	2 or more serving	Iron
dry beans and peas as		B-vitamins
alternates		
	4 or more serving, including	
	a dark green or deep yellow	
	vegetable at least every	
	other day.	
Vegetable-fruit group	A citrus fruit or other	Vitamins
	fruits or vegetable rich	Minerals
	in ascorbic acid- daily	Cellulose
	Other fruits and vegetables	
	including potatoes	
		Thiamine
		Niacin
Bread-cereals group	4 or more servings	Riboflavin
(Whole grain)		Iron Carbohydrates
ebrichesd restored)		Cellulose

The 4-food group plan.

The percentage of the Daily Recommended Allowances provided by the foundation pattern will vary with individual needs. The person with a greater requirement will have those needs less well satisfied, of course, than the person with a lesser daily need. A day's dietary planned with the use of the 4-food group is illustrated in table .

This menu contains more than the minimum number of servings in three of the four groups of plan (see Fig.). The nutrients contributed by foods in the four foundations groups in this dietary are shown in Table. Butter, jelly, mayonnaise, lemon pie, and sugar are not included in the calculations. A comparison of the percentage of the Daily Recommended Allowances provided by foods in the 4-group plan is made. Young men obtained a lower percentage of their allowance from the foundation groups simply because the recommendations for men are higher for some nutritents than for women. However, the young man, in satisfying his energy need and promoted by a natural urge to eat, selects more of all food groups. The result is that in actual practice the diets of young men are, as a rule, more nearly adequate than those of young women.

The 4-group plan is useful as an education tool to show the foundation for an adequate diet. Because it is such a simple plan, some may not realize its importance. For the most efficient use of the 4-group plan, one should know the main nutrients contributed by the various foods in each group.

The Nutritive Value of Food Commodities : Each food group, and each food within the group, makes a particular contribution to the nutrient content of the diet.

Comparison of the Nutrients Sulphide by the 4-Food Groups from the Above Menu to the NRC Recommended Daily Allowances for Young Women and Men

Young women (18-35 years)

Young men (18-35 Years)

Some foods supply many more of the nutrients and in much greater concentration then do athors. The nutritional contribution of the major food commodities, milk and milk products; meat, fish, and poultry vegetables and fruits; and cereal and cereal products, will be discussed in the following paragraphs.

Menu with the Four-Group Plan as a Guide

Breakfast		*Lunch*		*Dinner*	
Orange juice	4 oz	Swedish meat balls	3 oz	Veal cutlet	3 oz
Egg. soft-cooked	1	Green beans	½ c	Baked potato	1 med
w.w. toast	2 sl	Waldorf salad	2/3 c	Brocciol	2/3 c
Butter	1 pat	Pan roll	1	Hard roll	1
Jelly	1 tbsp	Cup custard	6 oz	Butter	1 pat
Milk, whole	8 oz	Iced tea	8 oz	Lemon pie	1 sl
		Snack -1 milk shake	Iced	tea	8 oz

Milk and Milk Products : Milk is considered as nature's "most nearly perfect food." Most of the known essential nutrients are found in milk, but it is a much better source of some than others. Milk and milk products are excellent sources of calcium, protein and riboflavin. Vitamin A, phosphorus, and thiamine are also supplied in good amounts. Milk and milk products are poor sources of iron and of ascorbic acid.

The importance of including milk or milk products in the diet so as to obtain sufficient calcium is well known. For students, or anyone for that matter, drinking milk is one of best ways of assuming an adequate calcium intake. Each gram of milk contains about 1 mg of calcium, with a glass of milk supplying about one-third of the recommended calcium intake for the college student.

Milk contains protein of high biological value; and so complements the incomplete proteins of cereal products, fruits, and vegetables. Since milk can very well be served as a beverage at each meal of the day, a source of complete protein can therefore be assured. The protein value of milk is that each ounce contains about 1 gm of protein.

Evaporated milk contains the same nutrients as whole milk. The process of evaporation, and pasteurization also, reduces the thiamine and ascorbic acid content by about one-fifth to one-fourth. Evaporated milk is convenient to use and economical.

The fortification of milk with vitamin D is a god public health measure. By adding vitamin D to milk the essential nutrients for bone formation, calcium, phosphorus, protein, and vitamin D, are brought together in one food.

Food	Measure	Energy, Cal.	Protein, gm.	Calcium, mg.	Iron mg.	Vit. A IU	Thiamine, mg.	Riboflavin, mg.	Ascorbic Acid mg.
Milk group									
Milk (beverage, custard, milk shake)	2½ C	400	22.5	720	0.3	875	0.2	1.05	5
Ice cream (shake)	1/8qt	145	3	87	0.1	370	0.03	0.13	1
	Total	*545*	*25.5*	*807*	*0.4*	*1245*	*0.23*	*1.18*	*6*
Meat group									
Egg, soft, ck,	1	80	6	27	1.1	590	0.05	0.15	—
Egg (custard)	1	80	6	27	1.1	590	0.05	0.15	—
Meat balls	3 oz	245	21	9	2.7	30	0.07	0.18	—
Veal cutlet	3 oz	185	23	9	2.7	—	0.06	0.21	—
	Total	*590*	*56*	*72*	*7.6*	*1210*	*0.23*	*0.69*	—
Vegetable-fruit group									
Orange juice	4 oz	50	.5	13	0.3	245	0.11	0.03	64
Green beans	1/2c	15	1.0	31	0.4	340	0.04	0.06	8
Apples	1/2c	35	tr	4	0.2	25	0.02	0.01	1
Celery	1/4c	4	tr	10	0.1	60	0.01	0.01	2
Potato, baked	1 med	90	3	9	0.7	tr	0.10	0.04	20
Broccoli	1/2c	20	2.5	66	0.6	1875	0.07	0.15	68
	Total	*219*	*7.0*	*124*	*2.1*	*2435*	*0.32*	*0.28*	*150*
Bread-cereal group									
Bread,w.w.	*2sl*	*110*	*4*	*44*	*1.0*	*tr*	*0.10*	*0.06*	*tr*
Roll,pan	*1*	*115*	*3*	*28*	*0.7*	*tr*	*0.11*	*0.07*	*tr*
Roll, hard	*1*	*160*	*5*	*24*	*0.4*	*tr*	*0.03*	*0.05*	*tr*
	Total	*385*	*12*	*96*	*2.1*	*tr*	*0.24*	*0.18*	*tr*
Grad total		*1734*	*100.5*	*1108*	*12.4*	*5000*	*1.05*	*2.35*	*169*

Table Nutritive Value of Milk and Some Milk Products

Milk and Milk Products	*Energy Cal.*	*Protein, gm.*	*Calcium, mg.*	*Irons mg.*	*Vit. A. IU*	*Thiamine, mg.*	*Riboflavin mg.*	*Ascorbic Acid, mg.*
Milk, whole (I c)	160	9.0	288	0.1	350	0.08	0.42	2
Buttermilk, cultured, skim (Ic)	90	9.0	298	0.1	10	0.09	0.44	2
Evaporated, water added (I c)	173	9.0	318	0.2	410	0.05	0.42	1
Cheese, process (I oz) 105	7.0	219	0.3	350	trace	0.12	0	
Chesse, cottage, creamed, skim milk (1/2 c)	120	15.5	106	0.3	190	0.03	0.28	0
Ice cream (1/8 qt)	145	3.0	87	0.1	370	0.03	0.13	1

Table Nutritive Value of Some Meat, Fish, Poultry, and Egg

Food	*Energy Cal.*	*Protein, gm.*	*Calcium, mg.*	*Irons mg.*	*Vit. A. IU*	*Thiamine, mg.*	*Riboflavin mg.*	*Ascorbic Acid, mg.*
Beef, round (3 oz)	165	25.0	11	3.2	10	0.06	0.19	0
Beef, liver, fried (3 oz)	195	22.5	9	7.5	45,200	0.22	3.55	23
Pork, lean and fat, loin roast (2 oz)	310	21.0	9	2.7	—	0.78	0.22	0
Chicken (3 oz)	170	18.0	18	1.3	200	0.03	0.11	3
Salmon (3 oz)	120	17.0	—	0.7	60	0.03	0.16	0
Egg (1)	80	6.0	27	1.1	590	0.05	0.15	0

Value depends on amount of bone consumed.

value. They provide protein and iron, with some phosphorus, thiamine, riboflavin, and niacin.

The popularity of non-fat milk solids is increasing because of the lower cost, ease of storage, and lower Calorie intake. With the removal of cream from the milk, which is done prior to drying, the caloric value is reduced by about one-half. In addition, vitamin A and other fat-soluble vitamins are removed. If nonfat milk solids are used to replace the whole milk, care must be taken to provide for additional vitamin A value from other sources such as green and yellow vegetables and liver because milk is depended on to provide some of the vitamin A need.

An ounce of Cheddar-type cheese provides about the same nutritive value as a glass of milk. In the manufacture of cheese some of the whey is removed, taking with it some of the water-soluble nutrients including lactose, the water-soluble vitamins (B-group), and minerals. Cottage cheese made with rennet has a higher calcium content than that made entirely by the souring of the milk (acid coagulation). In this process calcium, which is soluble in an acid medium, is carried into the whey.

Meat, Fish, Poultry, and Eggs : Meat, fish and poultry are very similar in their nutritive.

The protein in this group of foods, as in milk, is of high biological value. A 3-oz serving of meat supplies approximately 20 gm of protein, which is about one-third the Recommended Allowances for young adult women and over one-fourth for young adult men.

Iron is present in relatively high concentration in the organ meats, particularly liver and kidney, and in to a lesser amounts in muscle tissues. Meat is poor source of calcium . Some fish products, mainly shell fish and canned salmon, in which a portion of the bone is edible, are somewhat better than meat as a source of calcium.

Pork muscle is high in thiamine content whether other muscle meats contain only moderate amounts. The glandular organs, liver, kidney, heart, and tongue are higher than muscle meats in riboflavin content. Liver, the storage place for vitamin A, is only edible animal tissue containing any appreciable amount of this vitamin.

Eggs provide protein, iron, phosphorus, vitamin A, and riboflavin to the diet. The protein in egg, which is located both in the yolk and the white, is of good biological value. One egg contains about 6 gm of protein, approximately two-thirds the amount in one glass of milk. Phosphorus is distributed in both the white and the yolk. Iron and vitamin A are contained only in the yolk. Table gives the nutritive value of some kinds of meat, fish, poultry, and eggs.

Vegetables and Fruits : As a group, vegetables and fruits are the source of minerals, vitamins, and cellulose to the diet. Not to be disregarded is the interest they add because of their variety in colour, flavor, and texture. The great number of fruits and vegetables available for use differ markedly in nutrient content. For the sake of clarity they are grouped according to their contribution of nutrients to the diet.

Mostly the green and yellow vegetables and fruits are outstanding in their vitamin A values. One serving of sweet potatoes, carrots, kale or cantaloup furnishes sufficient vitamin A to meet the Recommended Allowance for vitamin A for persons of all ages. In addition leafy-green vegetables provide more calcium, iron , ascorbic acid, and the B-vitamins than other vegetables. Some of the green vegetables, spinach, chard, sorrel, and beet greens contain oxalic acid, which combines with calcium during digestion forming an insoluble salt that cannot be absorbed, and makes the calcium in those vegetables of no use to the body. However, these green vegetables, even though not supplying calcium, are invaluable in the diet for the generous amounts or iron, ascorbic acid, and vitamin A value they provide. The ascorbic acid content of broccoli, Brussels sprouts, kale, and similar vegetables is quite high.

Head lettuce, celery, cabbage, and other light green vegetables are important source for cellulose. Raw cabbage is a good source of ascorbic acid. The light green vegetables are low in vitamin A value.

Citrus fruits and tomatoes are good sources of ascorbic acid. Tomato juice contains about one-third as much as the citrus fruits.

Since they are available the year round and are well liked, it is customary to include citrus fruits in most dietary plans. Other foods like strawberries, cantaloups, kale, and green peppers are also rich in ascorbic acid as citrus fruits, but due to cost, unavailability, or lack of acceptance, do not fit into the diet as a routine item as well as citrus fruits. Ascorbic acid is easily destroyed during storage, freezing, and cooking. Citrus retain their ascorbic acid content better than other foods due to the preserving action of the acids they contain.

Vegetables of the seed, root and tuber classes, like Lima beans, corn green peas, sweet potatoes, and white potatoes are higher in carbohydrate content than other varieties. Starch is stored in these areas of the plant's structure.

Vegetables and fruits as a rule provide lesser protein, fat, and total Calories. Table shows the contribution of some fruits and vegetables to the diet.

Cereals and Cereal Products : Cereals are seeds of the grass family—wheat, corn, rice, oats, rye, and barley. From these cereal grains flours (whole wheat, white rye, barley etc.) are manufactured for the preparation of the many varieties of breads, cakes, pastries, breakfasts cereals, macaroni products, hominy corn sirup, corn meal, and other products. Whole wheat has the following composition in terms of grams of the constituent per 100 gm of whole wheat: 72 carbohydrate, 2 fiber, 12 protein, 2 fat, 2 ash, and 10 moisture.

In many countries cereals are the main food of the diet, furnishing 50 to 90 per cent of the total calories; in the United States about one-third of calories is from cereal or cereal products. More wheat and corn is grown in U.S.A. than other cereals; most of the wheat and corn is used for human consumption, a large part of the corn fed to livestock.

The cereal grains are easy to grow, easy to store, and have good keeping qualities. Whole grain cereals contribute calories (mainly in the form of carbohydrate), thiamine, iron, riboflavin, and partially in complete protein. Cereals are easy to digest, have a blend flavor, and supply roughage or cellulose.

Nutritive Value of Some Fruits and Vegetables

Food	*Energy Cal.*	*Protein, gm.*	*Calcium, mg.*	*Irons mg.*	*Vit. A. IU*	*Thiamine, mg.*	*Riboflavin mg.*	*Ascorbic Acid, mg.*
Apple (1 med)	70	tr	8	0.4	50	0.04	0.02	3
Banana(l med)	85	1.0	8	0.7	190	0.05	0.06	10
Broccoli, ck (1/2 c)	20	2.5	66	0.6	1875	0.07	0.15	68
Cabbage, ck (1/2 c)	18	1.0	38	0.3	110	0.04	0.04	28
Carrots, ck (1/2 c)	23	0.5	24	0.5	7610	0.04	0.04	5
Green beans, ck (1/2 c)	15	1.0	31	0.4	340	0.04	0.06	8
Kale, ck (1/2 c)	15	2.0	74	0.7	4070	—	—	34
Lettuce, Iceberg, (50 gm)	7	0.4	10	0.2	167	0.03	0.03	3
Lima beans, ck (½ c)	90	6.0	38	2.0	225	0.15	0.08	14
Orange juice, fresh (1/2 c)	50	0.5	13	0.3	245	0.11	0.03	64
Peaches, cn (1/2 c)	100	0.5	5	0.4	550	0.01	0.03	4
Potato, white, baked (1 med)	90	3.0	9	0.7	tr	0.10	0.04	20
Tomato juice (1/2 c)	23	1.0	9	1.1	970	0.07	0.04	20

Cereal and Cereal Products	Energy Cal.	Protein, gm.	Calcium, mg.	Irons mg.	Vit. A. IU	Thiamine, mg.	Riboflavin mg.	Ascorbic Acid, mg.	
Otameal, ck (1 c)	130	5.0	21	1.4	0	0.19	.0.05	0.3	0
Rice, white, enriched ck (1 c)	185	3.0	17	1.5	0	0.19	0.12	1.6	0
Macaroni, unenriched ck (1 c)	155	5.0	11	0.6	0	0.02	0.02	0.4	0
Macaroni, enriched ck (1 c)	155	5.0	11	1.3	0	0.19	0.11	1.5	0
Cake, plain (3 x 2 x ½)	200	2.0	35	0.2	90	0.01	0.05	0.1	0
Bread, white, unenriched (1 sl)	60	2.0	16	0.2	0	0.2	0.02	0.3	0
Bread, whole wheat (1 sl)	55	2.0	23	0.5	0	0.06	0.03	0.7	0
Muffin, enriched (1)	140	4.0	46	0.8	50	0.08	0.11	0.7	0
Biscuit, enriched									
(2 1/2" diam)	140	3.0	46	0.6	0	0.08	0.08	0.7	0
Pan roll, enriched									
(12 per Ib)	115	3.0	28	0.7	0	0.11	0.07	0.8	0

In the preparation of cereal products for the market, parts of the cereal grain are removed. In the case of brown rice only the outer husk is removed whereas in the preparation of white rice all of the outer coats are wheat flour is made from the entire grain except for the husk; white flour is just the endosperm portion. Most of the cellulose, minerals and B vitamins are in the outer layers or coats of the grain. The endosperm portion contains the carbohydrate and incomplete protein. The germ contains most of the fat of the grain and some of the thiamine. Because the fat tends to become rancid during storage and also seems to hold a great attraction for insects, the germ is usually removed in milling. Furthermore, the public prefers the refined product for mouses.

The protein in cereal products varies in biological efficiency but as a whole is classified as partially incomplete. However, with supplementation or protein from milk or meat or eggs, the cereal proteins make a significant contribution to the diet. About 20 per cent of the protein in diet is from cereal sources; on low-cost dietaries the percentage is relatively higher. Milk and cereal make a good nutritional team, cereal supplying iron, thiamine, and partially complete protein, and milk providing calcium, vitamin A, and complete protein. The use of the milk solids (dried milk) in bread improves the nutritive contributions of this product.

It is important that whole grain, restored or enriched cereals, and cereal products be selected for the diet in order to benefit from their greater nutritive contributions. Table gives the nutritive contributions of some cereal products to the diet.

Value of Energy

Energy for physiological activity is ultimately obtained from the sun. The sun gives out energy in the form of visible light waves and invisible ultraviolet rays. When these impinge on green plants, the latter are able to absorb the energy and build-up compounds and such as sugar and starch from the carbon dioxide of the air and the water of soil. The compounds become storehouses of energy within the green plants.

By the action of oxygen on these carbon compounds, they can again be broken down through a series of stages into carbon dioxide and water and, in the process, the stored energy is once more liberated. This breakdown happens in the plants themselves when they respire and is the source of energy used by them for growth, development and reproduction.

But far more energy is stored in starch and sugar than is used by the plants and, when animals eat the plant products, this energy becomes available to them.

Animals, too obtain oxygen from the air in breathing. This is transferred in the lungs to the blood and is carried to all parts of the body. Food which is eaten, digested and absorbed is also taken in the circulation to organs where it can be temporarily stored. Most of the starch and sugar eaten is stored in the form of another carbohydrate, glycogen, in either the liver or the muscles, and as we have seen, is broken down to provide energy.

The recognition of these facts led to a great deal of work on the quantities of food needed to produce the energy for certain tasks and it was found that the energy value of a food could be expressed in terms of a heat-unit or calorie. A calorie is the amount of heat-energy required to raise the temperature of 1 g. of water through 1 °C. This was found too small a unit to be convenient for expressing the energy values of foods, so a unit was chosen of 1,000 calories or 1 large Calorie (spelt with a capital C).

The next step was to find out how many calories were required by individuals of different weights, both resting and carrying out tasks with different energy requirements.

The following are average values:

	Calories
Metabolism of sleep (8 hours)	518
Basal metabolism while awake (16 hours)	1,152
Allowance for light work	1,200
Total	2,870

(Best and Taylor, 1950).

Daily Calorin Allowances for Adults

Requirement	*Description*	*Calorie requirement*
0	No work, almost basal (e.g. lying in bed).	1,750
1	Sedentary work (30 Cals/hr.) and little travelling (65 Cals.)	2,250
2	Light work (70 Cals. /hr.) and travelling (130 Cals.)	2,750
3	Medium work (100 Cals./hr.) and travelling (130 Cals.	3,000
4	Heavy work (200Cals. / hr.) and travelling (130 Cals.) Extremely heavy work (450 Cals./hr.) and travelling (130 Cals.)	5,000
0	No work, almost basal (e.g lying in bed)	1,500
1	Sendentay work (30 Cals./hr.) and little travelling (50 Cals.)	2,000
2	Light work (70 Cals./hr.) and travelling (100 cals.)	2,250
3	Medium work (100 Clas./hr.) and travelling (100 Cals.).	2,500
4	Heavy work (200 Cals./hr.))	
5	Very heavy work work(200 Cals./hr.) and travelling (100 Cals.)	3,750

The recognition that the quantity of food required could be exactly measured so captured the imagination that for many years no thought was given to the quality of the food supplied. Calories were all important and the neat way in which a man's energy needs could be expressed numerically no doubt delayed the recognition of the more subtle needs for particular factors in foods.

This is doubtless one reason why vitamins were not discovered until the present century, and why are still ignorant about certain aspects of nutritional requirements.

It is, however, established that the basal needs for calories, are best met by a balance between proteins, fats and carbohydrates: other needs are adequate amounts of fluid, certain mineral salts and vitamins.

Although this book is mainly concerned with vitamins, it is not possible to study them without reference to other nutrients.

The Table shows present-day views of human requirements of vitamins and calories.

The figures given in the table are, of course, averages. As with all physiological functions, there are great individual variations but these can be discovered only by experience. However, an example will serve to illustrate the point. Mr. A, a lean, bony man, has a hearty appetite and seems able to eat as much as he likes without showing any tendency to grow fat. By contrast Mr. B, who is also physically active, puts on weight without apparently eating to excess. These two seem to have different basal mechanisms for the use of food, one making his calories go further, as it were, than the other.

The same seems to be true, to some extent for vitamin needs. Among people in a group living on a diet deficient in one or other of the vitamins, some will show signs of disease, others, whose needs are evidently less, will escape.

Both nicotinic acid and nicitinatmide are physiologically active as what was originally the P-P factor. To avoid confusion with nicotine (which has no vitamin activity) the term Niacin was introduced in the U.S.A. and has been used in the table compiled by the B.M.A. Committee on Nutrition.

In planning diets, however, the table given can safely be used as a guide. Any individual idiosyncrasies in the nature of special needs must be allowed for separately.

Methods of Assessing the Adequacy of Diets : How can you assess that a diet which has been planned or eaten is adequate in nutrient content? There are various procedures for assessing the nutritive value of the diet. The most simple of these is the use of a "score card." The use of a food pattern as a guide in planning an adequate diet has already been discussed, and score cards have been developed for determining how well diet meets the

Vitamins in Nutrition and Health

Report of the Committee on Nutrition- B.M.A. 1950. p. 22 and p. 23 (extract)

Age and sex	Requirement class	Calories	Vit. A &- carotene i.u. daily	Vit. D i.u. daily	Thiamine mg. daily	Niacint mg. daily	Ribo flavin mg. daily	Vit. C mg. daily
Both								
0-1		1,000	3,000	800	0.4	4	0.6	10
2-6		1,500	3,000	400	0.6	6	0.9	15
7-10		2,000	3,000	400	0.8	8	1.2	20
Males								
11-14		2,750	3,000	400	1.1	11	1.6	30
15-19		3,500	5,000	400	1.4	14	2.1	30
	sedentary work	2,250	5,000		0.9	9	1.4	20
	medium work	3,000	5,000		1.2	12	1.8	20
	heavy work	4,250	5,000		1.7	17	2.6	20
Females								
11-14		2,750	3,000	400	1.1	11	1.6	30
15-19		2,500	5,000	400	1.0	10	1.5	30
	sedentary work	2,000	5,000		0.8	8	1.2	20
	medium work	2,500	5,000		1.0	10	1.5	20
	very heavy work		3,750	5,000		1.5	15	2.220
Pregnancy								
1st half		2,500	6,000	400	1.0	10	1.5	40
2nd half		2,750	6,000	600	1.1	11	1.6	40
Lactation		3,000	8,000	800	1.4	14	2.1	50

Vitamin B_1, aneurin and thiamine are synonymous but the most recent recommendation is that Thiamine should be adopted as the chemical name of vitamin B_1.

suggested pattern. A more precise method of evaluating the nutritive adequacy of diets is computing the nutrient content of each food using a food composition table. The most precise method of all is actual laboratory determination of the energy, protein, mineral, and vitamin content. The choice of the procedure for evaluating the energy and nutrient content of a diet depends on the use to be made of the findings and the accuracy with which the food consumption data were collected.

Use of Dietary Score Cards : Dietary score cards set up for evaluating the diet on the basis of food groups are used mainly as a basis for nutrition education programs (Tables). A limitation of each score card is its failure to give the complete nutritive contribution of each food. On the other hand, it is a commendable educational tool in that it encourages a varied diet and provides a good "rule of thumb" for the selection of an adequate diet.

Use of Food Composition Tables : By far the most common method of determining the nutrient content of the diet is the use of food composition tables. In various chapters of the book of the food tables have been used in the study of the energy value and content of the different nutrients of various foods. The values are obtained by laboratory analysis with each representing many determinations.

The composition of the same food varies widely, specially in fruits and vegetables. Growing conditions, variety, fertilizer treatment, care in handling, all make a difference. Preparation of the food for the table preservation, and storage also have an influence on the composition of most foods.

A Dietary Score Card

Foods	***Each Day You Need***	***Score for Your One Day Score***
Green and yellow vegetables (raw or cooked in small amount of water)	1 serving	10
Oranges, grapefruit, tomatoes, or other vitamin-C-rich food	1 serving	10

Contd...

Foods	*Each Day You Need*	*Score for Your One Day Score*
Potatoes and other vegetables and fruits	3 servings	5
Milk and milk products	Children, 3-4 cups Adolescents, 3-4 cups Adults, 2 cups	20
Meat, poultry, or fish	1 serving	15
Meat, poultry, fish, or meat alternates (dried beans, peas, peanut butter)	1 serving	10
Eggs	1 daily (at least 4 a week)	5
Cereal, whole grain or enriched	1 serving or 2 slices bread	
Bread, whole grain or enriched	1 or 2 slices at every meal	5
Butter or other fats	2 to 3 level tbsp butter or enriched margarine	5
A good breakfast, including some form of protein, as milk or egg		10
	Total	100

Those who have compiled food tables have had to decide on the values that they considered most representative for inclusion in the table. The necessity of exercising judgment in preparing a food table accounts for some of the differences that exist among the compilations of food composition values. As a rule the most food table includes new data add to the accuracy.

Short Methods Using a Food Composition Table : Short method for dietary calculation have been developed in which foods similar in composition are grouped, together, a representative value for each of the nutrients is calculated, and the values listed in a table. Totalling the amount of foods of like composition in a diet and computing the nutritive contribution of the group is shorter, of course, than computing each food separately. That is the manner in which the short methods save time in calculation.

The short methods are found to agree with the long or usual method if applied to a varied diet, and if the food habits do not differ widely from the usual pattern of the dietary habits of the people of a country as a whole. In regions where there is a relatively higher intake of certain foods, such as corn meal in the southern region, a revision in the cereal and bread portion of the table becomes necessary to obtain an accuracy approaching that of calculating each food individually. For survey studies the shorter method of dietary calculation has been found satisfactory. Time required for computation can be reduced without great sacrifice to accuracy.

Scientific Test

In research studies designed to determine quantitatively the nutrient intake as part of a metabolic balance study, the composition of a food is determined by laboratory analysis rather than by use of a food composition table Laboratory Analysis is the most accurate of any procedure for determining the nutritive value of food, since the nutrient content of some foods varies widely. To illustrate, the ascorbic acid content the thirteen different varieties of potatoes ranged from 8.2 to 17.4 mg. per 100 gm. of fresh weight, and for thirty-five varieties of cabbage from 32.4 to 100.7 mg. per 100 gm. of fresh weight. It should be recognized, however, that the fruits and vegetables vary more in composition than most other foods.

The differences between computed and analyzed values for given diets have been studied. It is generally concluded that agreement is sufficiently close to warrant the use of food tables in dietary surveys, reserving laboratory analyses for controlled studies.

Financial Restraints

Ultimately, daily menus, a market list, and a plan for purchasing food must be made by families who maintain households and by agencies who make allowances for families in need of assistance. The Consumer and Food Economics Research Division of the U.S. Department of Agriculture prepares materials that are of genuine assistance as guides in planning food budgets. The quantities and kinds of foods needed to adequately nourish different individuals are estimated at low-cost, moderate-cost, and more expensive diet. The Research Division has prepared plans for twenty age-sex groups and for eleven food commodity groups. These groups include milk and milk products; meat, poultry, and fish, eggs, dry beans, peas, and nuts; grain products; potatoes; citrus fruits and tomatoes; dark green and dark yellow vegetables; other vegetables and fruits; fats and oils; sugars and sweets.

To plan a food budget for a family of a certain size it is necessary to add together the estimated quantities needed for each family member. For example, a week's food plan for a family of a man and a woman both 33 years of age, a girl 8, and a boy 11 would be as summarized in Table.

The student of nutrition is aware that merely planning for kinds and amounts of food is not enough; the planning is made best with knowledge of the food preferences of the family and the availability and price of these foods. The budget plan allows for choice of foods within the commodity groups. Further adjustment can be made even between the groups with a knowledge of food values. For instance, potatoes could not substitute for eggs nutritionally, but another serving of meat would substitute very well.

The estimated cost of one week's food supply for a four-member family (a girl 8, a boy 11, man and woman each 33 years of age) as of January 1963 was $32.80 for the moderate-cost plan (Table).

It is gratifying that an adequate diet can be provided at different cost levels. The low-cost plan contains substantially more potatoes and grain products. The lower-cost meat cuts can be used in the limited-expense plan with the assurance that the nutritive value is equal to that of the higher-priced cuts. The moderate-cost and liberal plans include more milk, eggs, meat, fruits and vegetables. More expensive items such as foods out of season and the more highly processed foods are allowed in the moderate-cost and liberal plans.

Quantity of Food for a Family of Four for One Week

Food Groups	*Unit*	*Low-Cost Plan*	*Moderate Cost-Plan*	*Liberal Plan*
Milk, milk products	qt	16.5	17.5	19.0
Meal, poultry, fish	lb	11.5	17.2	20.8
Eggs	no.	25.0	29.0	29.0
Dry beans, peas, nuts	lb	1.4	.9	0.9
Grain products	lb	12.5	11.5	10.9
Potatoes	lb	10.0	8.5	7.8
Citrus fruit, tomatoes	lb	7.5	9.0	11.5
Dark green, deep yellow vegetables	lb	3.5	3.5	3.5
Other vegetables, fruits	lb	19.8	22.5	25.2
Fats, oils	lb	3.1	2.8	2.8
Sugars, sweets	lb	3.0	3.9	4.6

Cost of one Week's Food at Home[1] Estimated for Foods Plans at Three Cost Levels, June 1964, U.S.A. Average

Sex-Age Groups[2]	*Low-Cost Plan, Dollars*	*Moderate Cost Plan, Dollars*	*Liberal Plan, Dollars*
Families			
Family of two 20-35 years[3]	14.60	19.60	22.70
Family of two, 55-75 years[3]	12.20	16.50	18.70
Family of four, preschool children[4]	21.40	28.40	32.80
Family of four, school children[5],	24.60	33.00	38.30

Contd...

Sex-Age Groups[2]	*Low-Cost Plan, Dollars*	*Moderate Cost Plan, Dollars*	*Liberal Plan, Dollars*
Individuals[6]			
Children under 1 year	2.90	3.80	4.10
1-3 years	3.70	4.80	5.50
3-6 years	4.40	5.80	6.70
6-9 years	5.20	7.00	8.30
Girls, 9-12 years	6.00	8.00	8.90
12-15 years	6.60	8.80	10.20
15-20 years	6.90	9.00	10.20
Boys 9-12 years	6.10	8.20	9.40
12-15 years	7.10	9.70	11.00
15-20 years	8.30	10.90	12.60
Women, 20-35 years	6.20	8.30	9.40
35-55 years	6.00	7.90	9.10
55-75 years	4.70	6.90	7.80
75 years and over	4.70	6.20	7.20
Pregnant	7.50	9.60	10.80
Nursing	8.60	11.10	12.30
Men 20-35 years	7.00	9.50	11.20
35-55 years	6.60	8.80	10.20
55-75 years	6.00	8.10	9.20
75 years and over	5.60	7.80	8.90

Food Values and Food Costs : The buying of food is the largest single expense in the budget for most families. An average of 19 per cent capita of disposable personal income is spent for food in the United States. With increasing income, the per cent going food diminishes.

Economical purchase of food makes it possible to provide adequate diets at lower cost. Some nutrients are provided at less expense by one food or group of foods than by others. The approximate percentage of the food dollar spent for milk and milk products; meat, fish, poultry, eggs, dry beans, and nuts; vegetables; fruits; and grain products is shown in Fig. Other foods not included in Fig. are fats, sugar, and sweets, and miscellaneous items, which account for about 20 per cent of the total food expenditure. The protein group of foods is the most expensial, amounting to 37 cents of the food dollar or 37 per cent of the food expenditure. Milk and milk products account for 15 cents of the food dollar, vegetables 12 cents, grain products 11 cents, and fruits 8 cents.

Foods differ in the economy with which they provide the nutrients of the diet. Protein, calcium, vitamin A value, and thiamine were selected to illustrate this point. Using Fig. as a guide, in each food group if the nutrient bar exceeds the cost bar in length, that food group is a good buy for providing that nutrient, because the per cent of the expenditure for that group of foods is less than per cent of the nutrient obtained. The relative lengths of the bars will vary, of course, with price. It can be clearly seen that the milk group of foods is an excellent buy for calcium but only fair for supplying thiamine; the meat, fish, poultry, eggs, dry beans, and nuts group is a good buy for protein but a poor buy for calcium; vegetables are excellent for vitamin A, poor for protein; fruits are not a good buy for the nutrients listed, but had ascorbic acid been selected as one of the nutrients in the illustration, fruits would appear as good buy for that nutrient. Grain products are a good buy for protein and thiamine, and it may be surprising to note, for calcium, accounted for in part by the use of bread containing non-fat milk solids. Of course, little if any vitamin A value is furnished by grain products. The protein of cereals is economical to purchase and becomes of the good nutritional quality when supplemented with milk or other sources of complete protein. Grain products are a good buy for protein because, as shown in the cost bar is shorter than the protein bar.

3

Dietary Elements

Non-vegetarian Stuff

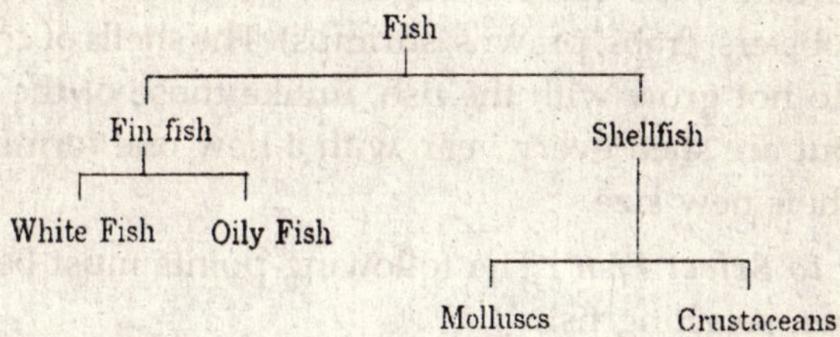

Fin fish are vertebrates and have skin and scales which cover the body. They move with the help of fins. They are subdivided into:

(1) *White fish* which are mainly flat fish, and contain oil only in the liver. Most of these are deep sea fish. Common local examples are pomfret, sole etc.

(2) *Oily fish* which are mainly round fish and contain fat all over the body. The amount of fat varies from 1.5% to 20% in different varieties. These fish are often pigmented and tend to be surface fish. Example: mackerels, sardines etc.

Shellfish, as the name denotes, have a shell covering the body. They are invertebrates. They are subdivided into:

(1) *Molluscs*: (a) Bivalves (e.g. oysters, scallops, mussels, clams and cockles) which have two distinctly separate shells joined by a hinge-like membrane. The movements of the shell are controlled by a strong muscle. When the muscle relaxes, the two halves of the shell fall open. The shell also opens when the organism dies, thus exposing the contents of the shell to contamination from outside, resulting in quick putrefaction. (b) *Univalves:* (e.g. whelks and winkles). These are recognized by the characteristic spiral formation of their shells, which unlike those of bivalves are not divided into halves.

The shells of molluscs increase at the rate of one ring per year to allow for the growth of the organism. The age of the mollusc can thus be roughly estimated by the number of rings on the shell.

(2) Crustaceans have a segmented, crust-like shell (e.g. lobsters, crabs, prawns, shrimps). The shells of crustaceans do not grow with the fish, unlike those of the molluscs, but are shed every year, with a new one forming to suit their new size.

How to Select Fish : The following points must be borne in mind when selecting fish:

(i) Eyes should be bright and not sunken.

(ii) Gills should be red.

(iii) The tail should be stiff.

(iv) The flesh should be firm and not flabby.

(v) The scales if any should be plentiful.

(vi) There should be no unpleasant odour.

(vii) To test a cut piece, press down with a finger, and if an impression is left then the fish is stale.

(viii) Any tendency for the raw flesh to come away from the bones is a dangerous sign.

Scaling and Cleaning :

(i) To scale, use the blunt side of the knife. Holding the fish by the tail, scrape firmly from the tail towards the head. Wash well to remove any loose scales,

(ii) Remove fins and trim tail,

(iii) To clean fish such as herrings, mackerel, etc., slit the belly, using a pair of kitchen scissors, from the head to almost half way down. Remove the head if desired,

(iv) In the case of flat fish such as pomfret, etc., cut away the gills, and make a small opening in the belly. Remove the entrails and wash well. If the head is to be removed, do this with a semicircular cut at the base of the head.

To Fillet the Fish: Slit the fish down the backbone with a sharp knife and separate the flesh from the backbone on each side with short sharp strokes. Then slit from the side and take out each fillet.

To Bone Herrings : After slitting and cleaning, open gently. Turn over and place the inside on hard board. Press firmly along the backbone to loosen the bone. Turn over and starting at the head raise the backbone with the thumb and forefinger. Pull the bone steadily away from the fish. After pulling out the bone, rinse the fish well and drain.

Cleaning of Fish

What to do	*What to do*
Do not work without having a basin prepared to hold the fish bones, and another one for the offal.	Wash and dry fish with a clean swab. Cut off all the fins and trim the tail; remove the eyes if necessary.
Do not work directly on a table; use a chopping board.	Remove the scales, if any, by scraping them with a knife from tail to head, then remove the gills.
Do not throw the fish scales on to the table; remove them from the knife by warping the knife against the side of the basin to collect them.	Remove all the entrails, roe, liver etc., from the gill-slits by pulling the gut out with a fork, or the hook of a small ladle handle. Make a small opening, 3½ to 5 cm. long,
Don't mix different fish together; always begin with one kind and place them on one side to be washed with the others, when they have all been cleaned from inside.	from the vent to the belly of fish such as herring, whiting, trout, and salmon, to remove the roe and clean the fish properly. For turbot, brill, etc. make the opening behind the head.

Contd...

What to do	*What to do*
Do not have your table covered with scales or offal of fish. Keep your chopping-board and table clean by swabbing often.	After removing roe, such as herring roe, place them immediately in a basin of cold water.
Do not forget, when removing the entails of a fish, to clear the bones of the blood vessels; and ensure that there is nothing left inside the fish by feeling with one finger.	If the head has to be removed, cut it from the gill in a V-shape.
Do not cut the ligament between the head and the body when removing the gills from small fish. Do not burst open or cut off the belly of a small fish when cleaning the inside	Wash the inside of the fish well under running cold water. With a clean or clothe swab or cloth dry inside as well. Then inspect the interior of the fish carefully.
Do not place a fish on a tray unless it has been well washed, dried and carefully examined.	

Cooking of Fish : The flesh of fish is very delicate and, therefore, great care must be taken to prevent the flesh from breaking during cooking. When boiling or cooking fish, the liquid should be at simmering point before fish is added as the connective tissue in fish is softer and the quantity is less than in meat. When preparing fish stew or fish curry, fish is put into cold liquid to flavour the gravy as well. Whole fish may also be covered with a cold liquid and brought to boil. This is done to prevent shrinkage of the skin. Steaming is a better method of cooking fish as it is a gentle method. Fish cookery is not a special method of cooking. All methods of cooking can be applied bearing in mind that the delicacy of the flesh of the fish and the fat content of the fish determine the cooking method. The time taken is always much less than for cooking meat. An average timetable is as follows, but much depends on the size and shape of the fish.

Boiling and baking	10 minutes per 500 gm and 10 minutes over
Steaming	15 minutes per 500 gm and 15 minutes over.
Stewing	Half to three quarter of an hour formes time the stew begins to simmer.

Frying		5 minutes
(for small fish or thin pieces)		
Grilling		5 to 7 minute's
Lean fish	Steamed or	Poached, deep-fried or baked in a
Oily fish	Baked	Sauce. Baked, grilled or pan-fried.

Boiling of Fish : Fish is generally boiled in a court bouillon. This is made of salt, water, milk and lemon juice for sea fish with white flesh. For salmon, trout and shellfish and various types of river fish the following court bouillon is used.

Court Bouillon

Water	1 litre
Salt	15 gm
Vinegar	75 ml
Carrots (sliced)	60 gm
Onion (sliced)	60 gm
Bay leaf	1
Parsley stalks	2 to 3
Peppercorns	6
Thyme	1

Simmer all ingredients for 30 to 40 minutes.

Strain and use as required.

The stock after fish is boiled can be used as a base for different types of sauces. Fish is cooked when the flesh separates easily from the bone. Test at the thickest part nearer the bone. It there is no bone then the fish is considered done when a creamy substance begins to run from the fish.

Steaming of Fish : Place the fish in a steamer. Sprinkle with salt and pepper. The water in the steamer must be fast boiling all the time the fish is cooking, if large, the fish can be turned once. Test as for boiling.

Grilling of Fish : Heat the grill and grease the rack. Clean fish. Sprinkle over with salt, pepper and lime juice. Gashes should be made on the fish to allow heat to penetrate, otherwise the outside becomes dry before the inside is cooked. For large fish, baste frequently with melted fat. For oily fish such as herrings and sardines, no extra fat is required.

Frying of Fish : Fish can be fried whole, if small, or cut into steaks or fillets or pieces if large. For cut pieces, it is preferable to coat the fish with egg and bread crumbs or seasoned flour and milk.

Baking of Fish : This method is most suitable for medium sized fish or the middle portion of a large fish. Scale and clean, but leave the head and tail on. Stuff the belly with a savoury forcemeat (11 gm fresh bread crumbs, 60 gm fat, grated rind of half a lime, 2 tsp chopped parsley, ½ tsp mixed herbs, salt and pepper and egg or milk to bind). Sew up with a needle and coarse thread. Do not fill the fish too tightly or it will burst, since the stuffing swells when it is cooked. Place the fish in a baking tray with a little fat, in a moderately hot oven, and cook till the flesh leaves the bones. To serve, remove the thread. Garnish with parsley and lemon. Serve with a sharp sauce.

Soused Herring or Mackerel : Soused herrings and mackerel are served as an hors d'oeuvre or for breakfast. Scale and clean the fish. Cut off the head and tail. Remove entrails. Wash well. Put back roe if any. Place on a plate. Sprinkle over with a little salt and leave for a couple of hours. Drain the fish. Roll up and place in a casserole dish. To 500 gm of fish add 12 peppercorns, 1 bay leaf and a large onion thinly sliced. Pour over equal proportions of vinegar and water, the liquid being just sufficient to cover the fish. Bring quickly to boil and simmer for a few minutes before removing from the casserole. Serve garnished with parsley.

Shellfish

Choosing Shellfish : They should be bought in season as far as possible. They should be medium- sized and of good weight. It is best to buy them' alive, particularly oysters, crabs, and lobsters. If they are dead, the following precautions must be taken: (a) The claws of crabs should be springy and not hanging down, (b) The eyes should be bright, (c) The tail of lobsters should spring back when stretched out. (d) Shrimps and prawns must be crisp, (e) Oyster shells should be tightly closed.

Preparing and Serving Shellfish : Shellfish can be served in a variety of ways. Lobsters and crabs are boiled alive. The meat is removed after cooking, flaked and replaced in their own shells with sauces or served in salads or other cold dishes. The meat is mixed with sauce and served in patties, or in scallop shells or on toast and canapes. Smaller shellfish such as prawns and shrimps must be shelled first, the intestines (the black thread- like substance found at the back) removed, then washed and cooked. They are served whole, boiled or steamed, stewed or in curries, fried with masala or in batter, devilled and in soups. Shrimps and oysters can be covered with sauces. Lemon and vinegar are served with shellfish to aid in digestion.

What to Serve with Fish

When fish is served as a main dish, it is usually served with potatoes, a salad or a cooked vegetable and a sauce. Here are some suggestions.

FISH	*POTATOES*	*VEGETABLES*	*ACCOMPANIMENTS*
Fried or grilled	Fried, boiled or sauteed	Green salad, cole slaw, green peas or beans, carrots, tomatoes parsnips, cauliflower,	Hollandaise, tartare, caper, tomato, mustard or cucumber sauces, lemon, parsley, butter, chutney, pickled beetroot or red cabbage.
Boiled or steamed	Boiled in jacket or mashed	Green peas or beans, carrots, tomatoes, spinach, celery, green salad, cucumber salad, parsnips, hot beetroot, sprouts, cauliflower, onions.	Hollandaise, cheese, horseradish, chutney, parsley, egg, fennel, anchovy or lemon sauces.
Baked	Baked, boiled or sauteed	Green peas or beans, carrots, green salad, tomatoes, cucumber salad, spinach, celery, parsnips, hot beetroot, sprouts, cauliflower, Onions.	Hollandaise, mustard, anchovy, cucumber, tomato, tartare, caper or brown sauces, lemon, parsley, butter.

Meat : The term meat is generally applied only to butcher's meat—beef, mutton, lamb, pork and kid.

The tenderness of the meat depends on the age and feeding of the animal, on the hanging and preparation after killing. Muscle structures have an effect on the tenderness and the texture of the meat. The skeletal muscles are made up of fibres which are composed of proteins, salts and nitrogenous extractives. The fibres are grouped parallel to each other in bundles held together by connective tissue and surrounded by a sheath of heavier connective tissue. The size of the bundles varies with different muscles and determines to some extent the texture of the meat. There are two kinds of connective tissue, collagenous or white connective tissue and elastic or yellow connective tissue.

The flavour of meat is determined by various factors such as feeding, age, sex and maturity. The older the flesh the greater the flavour in most cases; young flesh is not so highly flavoured but is sweeter and more tender. Flesh of male animals is stronger in flavour than that of females unless the animal has been castrated. Well developed muscles are usually more strongly flavoured, e.g., chicken leg as compared with breast. The longer the meat is hung the stronger the flavour, owing to certain chemical changes. Meat should not be eaten immediately after killing.

It has to be hung till tender. Shortly after death rigor mortis sets in and the muscles stiffen. Meat must be hung at 1° to 3°C (about 34° to 38°F) at least, till this passes off and until the acids which then develop have had a chance to soften the connective tissue. The enzyme present in the tissues also helps to make the meat render and more juicy. In cold countries this process takes at least 3 days but it is much quicker in warmer temperatures, varying between 12 to 24 hours. If so desired meat can be hung for a longer period. Not all meats should be hung like this and veal and pork particularly should be eaten fresh. They should also be thoroughly cooked before use.

Generally speaking, old meat and meat with considerable muscular development will be darker in colour and stronger in flavour. The flavour of the meat varies depending on the saltiness and sweetness of the blood, the species, the age and sex of the animal and the degree of maturity when eaten. Another factor is fat. Pork and mutton for example, have individual flavours depending on the fat. The third factor is the amount of sugar in the meat which on cooking tends to caramelize. Wherever possible select meat which is marbled. This is meat where the fat is interspersed between the muscle fibres and connective tissue. This shows good feeding. Marbling helps to keep the meat moist when cooked by dry methods. Marbled meat is also more nutritious.

There are no special methods of cooking meat and the fundamental methods of cooking can be deftly adapted to suit the particular joint. The amount of connective tissue present in the meat determines to a great extent the method of cooking. When connective tissue is present in large amounts, the meat, being tough, is cooked by moist methods. For those cuts which have only a small amount of connective tissue, dry heat cooking may be used. Long-fired cuts of meat require longer cooking than short-fired ones. They should be stewed or braised to make them tender. Shorter-fired meat is cooked by dry heat. The most developed muscle fibres are usually the longest and these coarser fibres are found in the legs, neck and tail. The shorter fibres are found in the fillet, rump and loin.

Dry heat cooking (roasting, frying and grilling or broiling) develops the characteristic meat flavour, coagulates the proteins, thus making fibres firm, hardens the connective tissue, and changes the colour. This change in colour is caused by a change in the composition of haemoglobin. Shrinkage is observed in meat cooked by the dry heat method. Moist cooking (braising, boiling, stewing, etc.) besides developing flavour and coagulating the meat, softens the collagenous tissue, thus rendering meat tender. Elastic connective tissue is softened only slightly by moist heat. There is no shrinking in meat cooked by moist methods.

When cooking meat it is desirable to retain the juices in the fibres. Steaks, roasts, etc., are cooked either at a constant temperature of 149°C (about 300°F) for beef, veal and lamb and 177°C (about 350°F) for pork, or by the searing method, where the meat is cooked at a high temperature for the first 10 minutes and then cooked at a lowered temperature. This method was supposed to help in retention of juices but this has been disproved although the aroma, flavour and colour that accompany searing are preferred by some. Steaks are usually grilled at 204.5°C (about 400°F). Studies have illustrated that a lower oven temperature 171°-177°C (about 300°-350°F) as compared to a higher temperature 218.3°-232.2°C (about 425°-450°F) results in less drip loss, less shrinkage, increased juiciness and more uniform colour throughout a cut. Overcooking or extended cooking at high temperature denatures the protein of meat, eggs, fish and birds or they toughen or become stringy or all three.

If a roast is cooked at a high temperature, the time of cooking is decreased, but dripping and evaporation losses are higher, and the meat is not so evenly cooked. The degree of 'doneness' also affects this loss, the steak done 'rare' or 'underdone' showing' less than that done 'medium' or Veil done'. A meat thermometer helps in determining the degree of 'doneness'. The thermometer should be inserted so that the bulb is at the centre of the cut but not in contact with the bone. For thin cuts the thermometer is not very satisfactory.

Meat meant for boiling should be dipped into salted boiling water and then allowed to simmer till tender. A pressure saucepan may be used to save time when cooking less tender cuts of meat. Care should be taken to prevent cooking of meat in a pressure cooker or at a high temperature longer than necessary, otherwise it becomes hard, dry and flavorless.

Frozen meat may be prepared by the same methods as fresh meat. It need not be thawed before cooking. If it is not thawed, however, the cooking time is considerably increased, to as much as two to three times the time required for cooking thawed or fresh meat. Thawing can be done in the refrigerator or at room temperature. When meat is not thawed, it does not retain a coating such as egg and bread crumbs.

Tenderisers such as papain (taken from raw papaya) may be used to soften the fibres before cooking. These must be applied to the meat, which should then be allowed to stand for one hour for a cut of 2.5 cm. (l") thickness. The acidity of vinegar, lemon juice, curd, cider and wine which can be added before or during cooking also helps to tenderise meat.

Sign of Quality : Mutton and lamb is meat from a lamb under one year old):

(i) A good quality animal should be compact and evenly fleshed,

(ii) The lean flesh should be firm, of a pleasing dull red colour and of a fine texture or grain,

(iii) There should be an even distribution of surface fat, which should be hard, brittle and flaky in structure, and of a clear white colour,

(iv) In a young animal the bone is pink and porous, so that when it is cut, a small amount of blood can be seen. With progressive aging the bones become hard, dense, white and inclined to splinter when chopped.

Order of Dissection :

(i) Remove the shoulders,

(ii) Remove the breasts,

(iii) Remove the middle neck and scrag end.

(iv) Remove the legs.

(v) Divide the saddle from the best end.

Approximate weight of the carcass of an Indian animal:

Lamb: 10 kg. (22 1b.)

Mutton: 16.8 kg. (37 lb.)

Whereas the approximate weight of an English animal is:

Lamb: 14 kg. (32 lb.)

Mutton: 23 kg. (50 lb.)

Pork

Fresh pork is at its best from September to April (the months with an 'r' in them). At 5 to 6 weeks it is known as suckling pig.

Sign of Quality

(i) Lean flesh should be pale pink, firm and of a fine texture,

(ii) The fat should be white, firm, smooth and not excessive,

(iii) Bones should be small, fine and pinkish,

(iv) The skin or rind should be smooth.

Joints and their Uses

	JOINTS		USES	APPROX. WEIGHT	
		French		(Lamb)	Mutton)
(i)	Shoulder	(L'epaule)	Roasting Stewing	2.00 kg	3.5 kg.
(ii)	Leg	(Le gigot)	Roasting Boiling	2.75 kg.	3.75 kg.
(iii)	Breast	(La poitrine)	Roasting Stewing	0.9 kg	1.75 kg.
(iv)	Middle neck	(Le collet)	Stewing	1.15 kg.	1.7 kg.
(v)	Scrag end	(Le cote decourverte)	Stewing Broths	450 gm.	0.9 kg.
(vi)	Best end	(Le carre)	Roasting Grilling Frying	575 gm.	20 kg.
(vii)	Saddle	(La selle)	Roasting Grilling Frying	1 kg.	3.5 kg.
(viii)	Kidney	(Le rognon)	Grilling Saute Braising	1.5 kg.	2.25 kg.
(ix)	Heart	(Le coeur)	Braising	115 gm	60 gm.
(x)	Liver	(Le foie)	Frying		350 gm.
(xi)	Sweetbread	(Le ris de veau)	Braising Frying		
(xii)	Tongue	(La langue)	Boiling Braising		

Pork : Fresh pork is at its best from September to April (the months with an 'r' in them). At 5 to 6 weeks it is known as suckling pig.

Sign of Quality :

(i) Lean flesh should be pale pink, firm and of a fine texture.

(ii) The fat should be white, firm, smooth and not excessive.

(iii) Bones should be small, fine and pinkish.

(iv) The skin or rind should be smooth.

1. Leg
2. Loin
3. Spare-rib
4. Belly
5. Shoulder
6. Head (whole)

   Trotters

   Kidneys

   Liver

Order of dissection:

(i) Remove the head.

(ii) Remove the trotters,

(iii) Remove the leg.

(iv) Remove the shoulder.

(v) Remove spare ribs.

(vi) Divide loin from the belly.

Joints and their Uses

	JOINTS *French*	*USES*	*APPROX. WEIGHT*
(i) Thigh	(La cuisse)	Roasting Boiling	4.55 kg.
(ii) Loin	(La longe)	Roasting Frying Grilling	5.45 kg.
(iii) Spare rib	(Le cote decou-verte de pore)	Roasting Pies	1.35 kg.
(iv) Belly (Breast)	(La poitrine)	Pickling Boiling	1.8 kg.
(v) Shoulder	(L'epaule)	Roasting Sausages Pies	2.7 kg.
(vi) Head (whole)	(La tete)	Brawn	3.6
(vii)	Trotters	(Le pied) Boiling	Grilling

Contd...

	JOINTS French	*USES*	*APPROX. WEIGHT*
(viii) Kidney	(Le rognon)	Saute Grilling	
(ix) Liver	(Le foie)	Pate	

Bacon and Ham : Bacon is made by preserving the meat of carefully bred pigs. The preservative used is salt. This can be applied in two ways:

(i) by covering the meat with dry salt and allowing at least 4 weeks penetration;

(ii) by using a sålt solution (brine).

This is injected into the flesh and then the meat is immersed in a salt solution for 5 days. Sometimes a combination of the two methods is used— brine is injected into the meat and the sides are then stacked and covered with dry salt for 2 to 3 weeks. It is then matured for about 3 weeks under controlled temperature. Desirable bacteria acting on the meat juices and salt produce the characteristics associated with well matured bacon.

This bacon is now ready for sale as 'green' or 'pale' bacon. In certain parts of the world the bacon is preferred smoked. So it is then hung over smouldering wood dust for 2 days. This extracts excessive moisture and gives the bacon a distinctive flavour. Smoking also improves the preservation as it acts as an antiseptic. This is particularly suitable in hot climates.

Good quality, well cured bacon should have a pleasant smell; the rind should be thin and smooth, the fat firm and free from any yellow marks, the lean part a good deep pink colour and the flavour mild and mellow.

1. End Collar
2. Prime Collar
3. Fore Hock
4. Top Back
5. Top Streaky
6. Back and Ribs
7. Prime Streaky
8. Short Back

9. Thin Streaky
10. Long Back
11. Flank
12. Corner Gammon
13. Slipper
14. Middle Gammon
15. Gammon Flock

Ham and Gammon : Ham and gammon come from the hind leg of a pig Gammon is cut off the side of a cured porker. Ham, on the other hand is cut off at the fresh pork stage and includes a substantial part of the loin. It is cured after cutting, usually by the long process of dry salting.

Cuts and their Uses

	CUT	*USE*
(i)	End collar	Boiling; Braising
(ii)	Fore hock can be bought boned and rolled	Boiling
(iii)	Prime collar	Boiling (either whole or cut into smaller pieces)
(iv)	Top streaky used for frying and grilling. Can be boned and boiled.	Thinly sliced rashers can be
(v)	Top back (good lean cut) in thin rashers and grilled.	Boiled or braised whole or cut
(vi)	Back and ribs	Cut into regathers and grilled.
(vii)	Prime streaky (the best cut of streaky bacon).	Boiled in one piece or cut into rashers.
(viii)	Short back (one of the best cuts for breakfast frying)	Frying
(ix)	Thin streaky Frying (Crisp and well cooked)	Grilling
(x)	Long back or grilled quickly.	Sliced thinly and fried gently
(xi)	Flank (good cut to be served with liver or other meats and in a minced bacon recipe)	Boiling Frying

Contd...

	CUT	USE
(xii)	Corner gammon (lean and well flavoured)	Boiling whole (serve hot or cut into rashers for grilling.
(xiii)	Slipper (gammon lean small cut)	Boiled whole or cut into rashers.
(xiv)	Middle gammon or lean rashers for frying.	Boiled whole (serve hot or cold)
(xv)	Gammon hock	Should be partly boiled and then baked (serve hot or cold.)

Beef

Signs of Good Quality :

(i) The lean meat should be bright red with small flecks of white fat.

(ii) The fat should be firm, brittle in texture, creamy white in colour and odourless. Older animals and dairy breeds have fat which is usually deeper yellow in colour,

(iii) Beef in good condition should have streaks of fat running through the lean section and the flesh should rise again quickly after being pressed with the fingers. Any cut surface should present a slightly moist appearance to the touch.

Order of Dissection : A whole side is divided into the forequarter and hindquarter, the division being between the wing ribs and fore ribs.

Hindquarter :

(i) Remove the rump, suet and kidney.

(ii) Remove the thin flank.

(iii) Divide the loin and rump from the leg. (The leg will consist of topside, silverside, thick flank and shin)

(iv) Remove the fillet.

(v) Divide the rump from the sirloin.

(vi) Remove the wing ribs.

(vii) Remove the shin.

(viii) Bone out the aitchbone.

(ix) Divide the leg into topside, silverside and thick flank.

Forequarter :

(i) Remove the shank.

(ii) Divide in half down the centres.

(iii) Take off the fore ribs.

(iv) Divide into joints.

Joints and their Uses

	JOINTS French	*USES*	*APPROX WEIGHT*
(i) Shin	Jambe de derriere (Jambe de devant)	Consomme beef tea, stewing	4.00 kg.
(ii) Topside	Culotte de boeuf	Braising, stewing, second-class roasting	7.5 kg.
(iii) Silverside	Gite a la noix, semelle	Salt beef	10.00 kg.
(iv) Thick flank	Gite a la noix	Braising and stewing	6.7 kg.
(v) Rump	Rump steak, colutte de	Grilling and frying as steaks or braised boeuf	7.2 kg.
(vi) Sirloin	Aloyau	Roasting, grilling and frying	10.00 kg.
(vii) Wing ribs	Cote d'aloyau	Roasting, grilling and frying steaks	5.9 kg.
(viii) Thin flank	Bavette	Stewing, boiling, sausages	4.00 kg.
(ix) Fillet	Filet	Roasting, grilling and frying	2.72 kg.
(x) Fore rib	Cote premiere	Roasting and braising	6.5 kg.
(xi) Middle rib.	Cote deactivate	Roasting and braising	8.00 kg.
(xii) Chuck rib	Cote du collier	Stewing and braising	4.08 kg.
(xiii) Sticking piece	Cou (collier)	Stewing and sausages	10.00 kg.
(xiv) Brisket	Poitrine	Salted and boiled	6.8 kg.
(xv) Plate	Plat de cot	Stewing and sausages	5.9 kg.
(xvi) Leg of	Gigot mutton	Braising and stewing	10.5 kg.
(xviii) Shank fat,	Jarret bone of kidney	Consomme, beef tea (trumeau)	4.08 kg. 7.2 kg.

N.B. : Weight of aitchbone x 10 = total weight of bones in hind quarter.

Minute Steak : Sirloin cut into 1.25 cm. (½")thick slices, flattened with a cutlet bat dipped in water to make the steak as thin as possible, trimmed and grilled or fried.

Sirloin Steaks: Sirloin cut into 1.25 cm. (½")thick slices, trimmed and fried or grilled.

Double Sirloin Steaks: Sirloin cut into 2.5 cm. (1") slices, trimmed and fried or grilled.

Porterhouse and T-bone Steak: Complete slices of sirloin including the bone and fillet.

Chateaubriand: This is a double fillet steak taken from the head of a fillet of beef, 3.5 to 10 cm. (1½"-4) thick, with an average weight of 340 gm. to 1 kg. It is generally served grilled at a temperature of 204.5°C (about 400°F), done to the taste of the customer.

Fillet Steak: These are approximately 115 gm. to 170 gm. in weight cut into 2.5 cm. (1") thick slices trimmed and grilled or fried.

Tournedos : Taken from the middle portion of the fillet. Remove all fat.

Fillet Mignon : Taken from the tail end of the fillet. All fat and sinews are removed and it is minced or sliced as required.

Entrecote Steak: A slice of steak cut between two bones of a rib of beef, or cut from the contrefilet (bone sirloin or undercut), and weighing about 650 gm.; sufficient for four persons.

Entrecote Minute: Cut as above from the sirloin or contrefilet as thinly as possible, about 1 cm. (2/5") in thickness, well flattened, and served grilled or sauteed.

Choosing Poultry : Only young birds are suitable for roasting; older birds may be boiled , steamed, braised or stewed. A roasting chicken should be about nine months to a year old; geese and other birds for roasting should not also be older than one year.

Signs of a Young Bird

(i) The feathers, especially the quills on the wings, should be easy to pull out.

(ii) There should be down all over the body, but especially under the wings.

(iii) No long hair on the body.

(iv) The skin should be white or clear and smooth.

(v) The feet should be supple, with smooth, even, overlapping scales,

(vi) The comb and wattle should be small and not well developed.

Signs which Show that a Bird is Fresh :

(i) Feathers - light and fluffy,

(ii) Eyes - prominent and clear.

(iii) No marked or unpleasant smell,

(iv) Feet - moist and not stiff and dry

(v) Skin - clear with no dark or greenish tinge.

Points which Denote Good Condition in Ducks : The breast should be plump. The bill and feet are yellow in young birds, but they darken with age. The webbing of the feet should be smooth, tender and easily broken, and the underbill soft and pliable.

Preparation

Storing Poultry: Fowls and ducks are best used fresh and should not be stored longer than 1 or 2 days before cooking. Protect them from flies and hang by the feet in a dry airy place.

Plucking : If poultry is plucked while still warm the feathers are easier to remove.

(i) When plucking, do not sit in a draught or the feathers will blow about.

(ii) Put the bird on a large sheet of strong paper.

(iii) Take care not to tear the skin, especially when plucking game birds.

(iv) Hold the bird firmly with the left hand and pluck with the right.

(v) Pluck out small handfuls at a time, starting from under one wing then continue plucking until one side is completely clear.

(vi) Remove all the pin feathers with a knife.

Singeing : A bird can be singed in either of the two following ways. Care should be taken not to scorch or blacken the skin.

(i) Hold the bird by its head and feet, and quickly and carefully singe off the hairs over a small gas jet.

(ii) Hold the bird in the left hand and singe with a lighted taper or paper spill.

The Giblets : These can be used for making stock for gravy to serve with the roast bird, for enriching the stock when the bird is boiled, or for making giblet pie or giblet stew. The liver and kidneys are not boiled with the fowl, as they tend to darken the meat. They may be half-cooked, chopped and used as part of the stuffing or cooked in other ways. Instructions for cleaning giblets are given below.

Liver: Carefully cut away the gall bladder, taking great care not to break it.

Stomach: Remove any fat and reserve it. Scrape the gizzard lining well.

Heart: Cut free of tubes, cut open, and scrape away all congealed blood.

Kidney: With a large bird, such as a turkey or goose, these are large enough to be used. Cut them open and cut out the core.

Neck: Scrape away all congealed blood.

Wash the liver, gizzard, heart, kidney and neck in salt water and rinse well.

Drawing the Tendons : If a bird is not young and tender, it is advisable to draw the tendons from the legs before roasting.

(i) Carefully cut through the skin of the leg at the knee joint, taking care not to cut the tendons at the same time,

(ii) Break the joint and swing the leg free to expose the tendons,

(iii) Pull out the tendons one at a time with a strong metal skewer. There will be 7 of them in each leg.

Stuffing : Birds can be roasted, stuffed or unstuffed, but they are usually stuffed. Stuffing can be put inside the bird only, or both inside and at the crop, covered by the skin of the neck.

Veal forcemeat may be used for the inside and sausage meat for the crop or vice versa. Pack the veal forcemeat, or any similar stuffing, fairly loosely to allow for swelling.

Trussing :

Method (A)

A trussing needle and some thin, clean string will be necessary. A trussing needle is a strong steel needle about 23 cm. (9") long with a large eye.

(i) Fold the skin of the neck over the back of the bird, and cross the tips of the wings over, to keep it securely in position.

(ii) Turn the bird breast upwards and put the tail through the vent.

(iii) Thread the trussing needle and pass it just under the top joint of the right wing through the bird and out through the same joint in the left wing. Run the needle back through the bird so that it enters and comes out just above the bottom joint of the wings.

(iv) Tie the ends of the string securely in a bow, taking care not to drag the flesh.

(v) Re-thread the needle, press the legs well into the sides towards the wings, plumping out the breast, and run the needle through the back of the bird, just under the thigh joint, and return through a point near the ends of the legs. Tie both ends of the string firmly together.

Method (B)

(i) Fold the skin of the neck over the stuffing and secure firmly with a small skewer.

(ii) Turn the bird breast upwards and put the tail through the vent.

(iii) Pass a large skewer through the wing pinions to hold them securely in position,

(iv) Tuck the legs well into the sides of the bird to plump out the breast, then tie the legs firmly together with a string; pass the string underneath the bird, cross it, then bring it up again and twist it round the wing. Skewer and tie firmly.

Trussing a Fowl for Boiling :

(i) Cut the skin of the legs all round at the knee joint, crack the joints and pull the shanks off with as many of the sinews as possible.

(ii) Thread the trussing needle and secure the wings in the same way as for the roasting bird, or fix them securely with a skewer,

(iii) Carefully loosen the skin round the legs, and slip them into the body of the bird. Secure in position with the trussing needle and string or with a skewer.

Vegetarian Stuff

Test for Freshness : All vegetables, particularly green ones, are best when taken straight from the garden. But this is not always possible so it is essential that one should know how to judge a well-grown vegetable. A well-grown vegetable is usually tender and free from pests.

Vegetables are classified into three divisions: (i) Root vegetables, (ii) Leafy vegetables, (iii) Other vegetables grown above the soil.

Root Vegetables : These should be firm and heavy for their size. They should be free from earth and grubs. Carrots should be heavy, smooth skinned and orange in colour.

Leafy Vegetables : These should be crisp and give a crunchy sound when squeezed. Break the vein of a leaf; it should give a sharp snap. It the leaves are limp, then the vegetable is not fresh.

Other Vegetables : Cabbage and cauliflower should be free from greenfly. The cabbage should have a firm heart and the outer leaves should stand the same test for freshness as green leafy vegetables. Cauliflower should have a close, white flower. Tomatoes should be of a rusty red colour and should not be soft. Runner beams and French beans should not be stringy. Peas should be full in the pod, and green. Ladies fingers should snap if the ends are broken. Brinjals should have a smooth skin and should not be heavy for their size.

Valued Food

Vegetables play an important role in the human diet. Properly chosen and eaten, cooked or raw, they make an invaluable contribution toward the supply of vitamins and minerals. Root vegetables are good sources of carbohydrates, and pulses (peas, beans, lentils, etc.) of vegetable proteins. A good balance of ingredients essential for growth and maintenance in human beings is more easily attained by a diet made up of both plant and animal life. Vegetables also provide variety in a meal, help to make a meal attractive by introducing colour, and furnish roughage.

Mushrooms have been found to contain one or more antibiotics, one of which is effective against tuberculosis and germs which cause boils. Mushrooms which have always been a food favourite are rich in vitamins and low in calories. Seven average sized mushrooms have only 1-2 calories.

Whenever possible at least two vegetables should be served in addition to potatoes. Salads should be made popular and should be served at both meals.

Salads are dishes made up of meat, poultry, game, fish, shellfish, eggs, vegetables, fruits and milk products—normally served cold but can be served hot or frozen. They can be made out of a single ingredient or a combination of ingredients. Salads are normally served as an accompaniment to the main course, a meal by itself or a sweet course (dessert). There should be special stress on hygiene as most of the ingredients are served raw. The ingredients used and the colour, flavour, texture and presentation may be varied according to the purpose.

There are four basic parts in a salad:

The Underliner : These are generally greens either shredded or in large pieces. Tear the greens instead of cutting with a knife. The greens must be crisp and chilled. To keep the greens crisp, it is necessary to store them in a manner that retains the maximum amount of water in the cells. This could be achieved by storing them at refrigeration temperature in the hydrator drawer wrapped in a moist cloth or in a covered container. The loss of water in cells can be reversed. To do this reduce the temperature to 2-3°C (about

34°F), and moisten the greens. When the cells are once again filled with water the greens will be crisp.

The Body or Heart of the Salad : This will form the major component and can be made of one ingredient or a combination of ingredients. Ingredients should look sparkling fresh with each individual piece intact. Fruits are particularly fragile and should be handled as little as possible. Dressings These make the salad more appetising although diet conscious people today eat their salads without a dressing.

Dressings : Dressing must be carefully selected. Depending upon the salad, the dressing could be either basic French or an emulsion. Pleasing flavours can be added to and variations made in the dressings by adding ingredients like cayenne pepper, tobacco sauce, diced hard boiled eggs, assorted herbs, a variety of cheeses, chutney, etc. Dressings should enhance the salad and not obscure it.

Garnish : The garnish should be the focal point and should be carefully selected for its simplicity and to enhance eye appeal and flavour. Edible garnish is more appropriate than inedible ones. Sometimes the dressing is also used as a garnish by piping it in a decorative form on the salad.

Special stress should be given to the quality of ingredients, eye appeal, simplicity, neatness and contrast or harmony in colour and in texture. All ingredients should be edible, clean, fresh and free from defects, such as bruises, rotten spots, insects, dirt, sand and insecticide. Raw fruits and vegetables should be at their optimum stage of maturity. All inedible Portions should be removed. Remove any excess moisture from ingredients as it thins the dressing, making it less effective.

The aesthetic qualities are determined by the form and shape of the food as well as by the colour. Skilfulness and artistic cutting and arranging of salad ingredients can create an appealing effect.

Try for an uncluttered appearance.

Always prepare salads as close to time of serving as possible.

They should be washed before peeling. A knife or a peeler may be used.

The purpose of cutting is to ensure uniformity of size and even cooking.

The types of cutting used for vegetables are dicing, chopping, grating, slicing, shredding, cutting into rings, mincing, etc. The object of preparation is to remove spoilt, soiled and indigestible parts.

Cooking : Fruits and vegetables are cooked for many reasons:

(i) To preserve them,

(ii) To soften the product,

(iii) To improve the flavour.

(iv) To increase the digestibility.

Whatever the methods of cooking applied, the objective is to lose as little as possible of the natural flavours, colour and nutrients.

Cooking affects the palatability of the vegetables, i.e., their texture, flavour and colour. While palatability may not affect the nutritive value of vegetables, it affects their desirability.

All the different methods of cooking can be effectively employed in the preparation of vegetables.

The effect of cooking on starch, protein and cellulose brings about the change in texture observed in vegetables when they are cooked. The predominant cause for change in texture will depend upon the composition of the vegetable. For example, with leafy vegetables which contain a high percentage of fibre, the change in texture is primarily due to the effect of cooking on the hemicellulose, whereas in potatoes the gelatinization of starch is the chief factor. While this is true, it has also been noted that the change in any one ingredient is not the only cause that makes vegetables tender. For example, gelatinization of the starch in a potato is completed before the potato is considered done.

As the amount of protein in vegetables is small, the effect of coagulation during cooking is not of great significance.

Alkalies such as baking soda aid in softening of vegetables as they speed up the solution of pectic substances and dissolve the hemicellulose. Acids, on the contrary, harden the vegetables, as acid precipitates pectin.

The texture of the cooked vegetables can be controlled to a great extent by the length of the cooking time. The longer the cooking period, the softer the product.

Flavour : The flavour of vegetables depends upon many substances—sugar, acids, tannings and a variety of volatile substances. There is a predominance of sweetness in beetroot, peas, corn and carrots, but each vegetable has other ingredients which contribute to its characteristic flavour and aroma. The pronounced bitterness or astringency of certain vegetables is due to the presence of tannin. The characteristic odour of the onion family—chives, shallots, onions, garlic and leek—is due to a readily volatile substance—allyl propyl disulfide. As this substance is soluble in water the longer the vegetables are cooked in water, the milder is the flavour.

The colour of the cooked product will depend on the kind and amount of colour pigment, the method of cooking and the acidity of the cooking medium. The colour pigments of fruits and vegetables are chlorophyll, carotenoids, flavones and anthocyanins. Tannings, though not colour pigments, undergo chemical changes during cooking and thus affect the colour of many cooked vegetables.

Chlorophyll : Chlorophyll is made up of two compounds, chlorophyll 'a' and chlorophyll 'b'. Both are organic esters and both contain magnesium. The reactions taking place during cooking affect these radicals. Chlorophyll is slightly soluble in water but dissolves easily in many organic solvents. Like other esters it is subject to hydrolysis, the reaction taking place in the presence of alkali, forming chlorophyll liens—salts of chlorophyll which are intensely green in colour.

In the presence of acids, chlorophyll undergoes another type of decomposition with the loss of magnesium from the molecule. The resulting compounds are called phaeophytins. They are yellow to brown in colour. Both reactions, with acids and with alkalis, are irreversible in the sense that chlorophyll cannot be formed again by treating the decomposed products with a neutralizing agent.

Any cooking process which involves the use of acids or alkalies will affect the colour of green vegetables. During the life of the plant the chlorophyll is held in the cytoplasm of the plant cells in such a way that it is protected from the regions of changing acidity. When cell life is destroyed, the constituents of the cells intermingle and the green colour fades, becoming yellow and brown.

When a green vegetable is cooked the cell structure gets slowly destroyed and the acid of the cells gradually comes in contact with the chlorophyll. Hence green vegetables cooked for long periods lose their greenness. If the cooking pan is kept open during cooking, some of the acids of the vegetables may evaporate, preserving some of the green colour. When soda is added to the water in which green vegetables are cooked there is no loss in colour. The alkali neutralizes the acidity of the vegetable and also speeds up the cooking process. Loss of colour also depends on the temperature of cooking. At high temperatures there is greater hydrolysis and, therefore, greater loss of colour.

Carotenoids : Carotenoids include two types of colour pigments—the hydrocarbons, e.g. carotene as in carrots, and the oxygenated hydrocarbons, e.g. lutein, the colouring matter in egg yolk.

These pigments like all other hydrocarbons do not dissolve readily in water. They are also not affected by acids or alkalies. The oxygenated carotenoids are also chemically resistant to acids and alkalies as well as insoluble in water. Other carotenoids are xanthophyll, associated with carotene, lycopene (the red pigment in tomatoes and watermelon), zeaxanthin (the yellow pigment in egg yolks and corn), capsanthin (in red pepper) and fucoxanthin (in brown seaweed).

Anthocyanins : Anthocyanins are colour pigments which are found more in fruits and flowers than in vegetables. The colour varies from red to blue. Red or purple cabbage, purple broccoli, beets and skins of aubergine and radish contain large amounts of anthocyanins. There are 28 known anthocyanins. They differ in their degree of solubility and sensitiveness to conditions which produce colour changes. They are inclined to be red in acidic and blue in basic solutions. The colour changes of anthocyanins, unlike those of chlorophyll, are reversible.

While cooking vegetables containing anthocyanins, the loss of colour as well as change of colour must be considered. Beets lose their colour or 'bleed' during the preparation. This is due to the great solubility of anthocyanins. High temperatures bleach this pigment, the colour returning partly when it is cooled.

Natural acids in fruits increase the redness of the cooked fruit. The colour of cooked red cabbage depends on the acidity of the cooking water. Tap water gives it a purple colour. Red cabbage is produced by adding acid to the water. The addition of cooking soda gives a bluish product.

Flavones occur in all plants, but particularly in white onions, white cabbage, cauliflower, etc. In an acid medium, they are colourless, while in a basic medium they are yellow. The reaction like that of arithocyanin, is reversible. Vegetables such as cauliflower can be made to change colour from white to yellow and back by holding them in fumes of acid or ammonia. Flavones are readily soluble in water as can be observed from the colour of the alkaline vegetable water, which is yellow. During cooking it is important to see that white vegetables do not turn yellow. The addition of acids such as lime juice or vinegar will keep them white.

Boiling : Vegetables are usually put into boiling liquid. This is to prevent the nourishment escaping into the liquid and also to curtail the action of plant enzymes which have harmful effects on vitamins. The exceptions to this are dried vegetables and root vegetables which should be started in cold water. Salt is generally added to the water, except when cooking dry vegetables, which do not cook well if salt is added at the commencement. The lid is kept on generally, except when cooking green vegetables, where the volatile acids present in chlorophyll must be allowed to escape or else they will discolour the vegetables. Lime juice brings out the whiteness of cabbage and cauliflower if added before cooking.

Potatoes : Scrub and scrape new potatoes, peel and eye old ones. Keep under water to avoid discolouration. To boil, put in salted water and cook till tender, drain and use as required.

Roast Potatoes : Parboil, drain and cook in dripping around the meat for at least 45 minutes.

Saute Potatoes : Slice cold boiled potatoes and fry in very little fat till brown.

Potato Chips : Two methods are used:

(i) Peel and cut them in to finger lengths. Parboil, drain and put into hot fat. Remove when half done. Put into smoking fat or boiling fat and brown just before serving.

(ii) Cut the peeled potatoes into finger lengths. Dry on a towel. Deep fry in a pan till a faint blue smoke rises. Fry chips until golden brown. Drain on absorbent paper, add salt.

Spinach : Remove the stalk and damaged leaves. Wash very thoroughly in several batches of water to remove grit and mud. Put into a pan. Add salt. Place over gentle heat, when the juice begins to run over spinach, raise temperature and boil for 15 minutes. Drain and chop or sieve as required. Add pepper and a small knob of butter to taste.

Before cooking spinach and other leafy vegetables, soak them for some time in water to which a little sugar has been added. This improves the flavour.

Green Peas : Shell peas and place in boiling water with ½ teaspoon of sugar, salt and a sprig of mint. Boil till tender. Drain. Take out the mint and add a little butter.

French Beans : String the beans. Slice them diagonally and cook in boiling salted water till tender (approx. 20 minutes). Cook with the lid off. Drain well and add a knob of butter.

Brussels Sprouts : Found in a temperate climate. Cooked the same way as cabbage but kept whole. Slit stalk end into four before cooking.

Cabbage : Wash well, remove coarse leaves but use dark outer leaves. Cut in half. Remove the hard centre stalk, shred. Cook in a little boiling and salted water till tender (10 to 15 minutes approx.). Drain well. A few bacon rinds can be added to the water. Serve plain or tossed in melted butter.

Cauliflower : Wash thoroughly, remove outermost leaves if necessary but leave some on. Turn over and cut across the stalk.

Put the cauliflower into boiling salted water and cook for 20 to 30 minutes.

Broccoli : Three types—white, green and purple.

Purple and green: To prepare, remove coarse stalks and wash the leaves and sprigs. Boil. Serve same way as cabbage or cauliflower. Particularly good with white saxice.

White: Prepare and cook as for cauliflower.

Turnips : Peel rather thickly. Cook in boiling salted water till tender; this takes 20 minutes to one hour. Drain, add white pepper and salt and butter. The cooked turnips can also be mashed up.

Vegetable Marrow : Very young vegetable marrow may be boiled whole and unpeeled. Cook in salted water for 15 minutes. Drain and serve with melted butter. Large marrows must be peeled and the seeds removed. Drain well and serve sprinkled with brown bread crumbs or with cheese sauce. Marrow may also be baked whole, (peeled or not) and stuffed with any savoury filling. Bake in a moderate oven at 177°C (350°F) for one hour. Cover the marrow with greased grease-proof paper.

Onion : Remove the root and the outer skin. Apart from being used as a flavouring agent, onions can be boiled and served as a vegetable or used stuffed.

Tomatoes : Grilled, fried, stewed, baked or raw.

Carrots : Scrub and scrape lightly. Peel old ones. Cut into strips or into roundels. Add just enough water, salt and a little butter. Cook till the carrots are tender and the water has evaporated. Serve sprinkled with chopped parsley. Young carrots can be boiled whole.

Corn on the Cob : Remove the sheath and silk threads. Cook in salted, boiling water till tender. Serve with melted butter.

Sweet Pepper : Capsicum, red or green. This can be served cooked or raw. To prepare the pepper, wash, cut out the stalks and remove the seeds. Red and green peppers may be cooked together to make a colourful vegetable dish. Slice and cook in a little salted water. Add a knob of butter. They may also be served stuffed, baked, boiled or stewed.

Celery : Wash celery thoroughly, using a brush to remove all soil. Separate the stalks. Tie into bundles. Cook in boiling salted water till tender. Drain and serve with white sauce.

Beetroot : Cut out the stalks about 2.5 cm. (1") from the root, taking care not to damage the skin. Wash and boil in salted water till tender (about 2 hours). Peel off the skin. Cut into cubes or slices and either serve hot, coated with white sauce, or cold in vinegar.

Leeks : Remove the coarse outer leaves. Cut out the roots and green top. Split the leaf end so that it can be washed thoroughly. Tie in bundles and boil in salted water. Drain. They are usually served with white or cheese sauce.

Broad Beans : Shell the beans. Cook them in boiling salted water and drain. Serve with parsley sauce. Skin older beans before serving.

Parsnips Peel thinly, using a potato peeler. Cut as required. Boil or bake.

Asparagus : Cut the woody portion, scrape the white part lightly. Remove any coarse spine. Tie in bundles. Place upright in a pan of salted water and boil for 10 minutes. Then lay the asparagus flat and cook till tender. Drain well, remove the string and serve with melted butter.

Artichokes : Only the lower parts of the leaves and lower sections are edible. Wash well. Cut off the stems and trim lower leaves if necessary. Place head downwards in boiling salted water and boil gently until tender, for about 30 minutes with the lid off. When cooked, the leaves should be easy to pull off. They may also be dipped in a thin batter and fried. Serve hot with melted butter or margarine or hollandaise sauce. Do not pour the sauce over the artichokes. The lower sections without the leaves may also be used, either raw or cooked, in salads.

Artichokes (Jerusalem) : Scrub well, peel, and to keep them white until ready to be cooked, place in a bowl of water to which a little vinegar has been added. Boil or bake. Serve plain boiled in the same way as potatoes or with white sauce. A very good au gratin can be made with these artichokes. Can be served in soups, separately or with another vegetable such as celery.

Colour Reaction of Vegetable Pigments

Pigment	*Vegetable*	*Colour in acid*	*Colour reaction in alkali*	*Colour reaction to metals*
Flavone	Cauliflower	Colourless (white)	Yellow	All-yellow Iron-brown
Anthocyanins	Red cabbage Beetroot	red	blue to green	Iron-blue Tin-purple
Carotenoids	Carrots	orange	orange	
Chlorophyll	French beans Spinach	olive green	bright green	Copper-bright Iron-green

Pulse

Nutritive Function : Pulses are a good source of vegetable proteins and vitamin B complex. Being substances with very little taste, they should be combined with spicy and strong foods, e.g. bacon, ham, etc.

In Western preparations pulses are combined with onion, tomatoes, leeks, celery and bacon rind.

In Indian preparations pulses are combined with spices, coconut milk, tomatoes, leafy vegetables and herbs.

Cooking :

(i) If with skin, soak overnight in boiling water to soften skin, e.g. haricot beans, thick peas, etc.

(ii) Wash first before soaking so that the pulses can be cooked in the same liquid in which they are soaked. Those with no skins like lentils can be soaked in cold water. Bring to boil and cook with lid on.

(iii) Add salt after cooking, as salt inhibits the normal cooking process of lentils and pulses. Those with skins can be made into a puree, as it is the skin that causes indigestion.

In Western preparations these foods are rarely served plain boiled. They are generally mixed with other foods and browned by baking or frying. Use liquids for soups and gravies.

Cheese : Cheese, one of the oldest known food products, is universally popular. The chemistry involved in changing semifluid milk into semisolid cheese is complex and many factors enter into the final curing of cheese to produce the different varieties but they all begin with the action of rennet or lactic acid which performs the same basic function, that of coagulating the milk proteins. Simply defined, cheese is the solid or casein portion of milk separated from the whey. The curdling of the casein is brought about by the action of rennet or lactic acid. The many different cheeses are the result of variation in the making and curing of each variety after initial curdling has taken place.

Many experiments and inventions in many countries of the world have produced cheeses ranging in texture from very soft to very hard and in flavour from extremely mild to very sharp. These cheeses are known by thousands of names, generally with names taken from the localities where they were first made.

***Classification*:** Cheeses are classified into large general groups according to whether they are started by the rennet or lactic acid method. They may also be classified as unripened, mould ripened and bacteria ripened or as soft cheese, hard pressed cheese or blue veined cheese.

Cheese is one of the most highly concentrated of all protein foods. It is also readily digested. Experiments have shown that from 90 to 99% of all cheese is digested. It is also a complete protein. Since approximately 10 litres of fluid milk are required to make 1 kg. of cheese, cheese contains many of the nutrients of milk in highly concentrated form—milk proteins, fat, fat-soluble vitamins and minerals.

Wholemilk cheese contains the same properties as milk. Certain cheeses such as blue veined are made out of skimmed milk and, therefore, are less nutritious.

Normally cow's milk is used to make cheese, but certain well known cheeses are made from goat's milk. The texture of the cheese from goat's milk differs slightly from that of cow's milk. It is more crumbly. Sheep's milk can also be used. The quality of the cheese depends to a great extent on the breed and the condition of the animal and the fodder given to it. Cheshire cheese is said to owe its fine flavour to the wild radish on which the cows feed, and its special nature is due to the mineral in the soil. Cheshire cheese, therefore, cannot be made in any other place as cheddar cheese can.

Certain cheeses develop a blue vein in maturing. This is sometimes a purely natural development, often sporadic and unpredictable. Sometimes fresh cheese is inoculated with pieces of blue cheese to catch the mould by contact. In some cases special bacilli are introduced. The mould is sometimes strengthened by brushing the cheese clean while the skin is soft, dipping it in whey and then rubbing it slightly with butter. This is done once a day for 10 to 20 days. Sometimes cheese is pierced with a copper wire. The main classes of cheese are:

(i) Unripened soft cheese, e.g. Cottage cheese, Cream cheese, Neufchatel.

(ii) Ripened in moulds by bacteria, e.g. Brie and Camembert.

(iii) Ripened by bacteria, e.g. Limbourger.

(iv) Semi-hard, ripened by bacteria in moulds, e.g. Gorgonzola, Roquefort and Stilton.

(v) Semi-hard, ripened by bacteria, e.g. Brick cheese, Munster.

(vi) Very hard cheese without gas holes, e.g. Cheddar, Edam, Gouda and Cheshire.

(vii) Very hard cheese with gas holes, e.g. Gruyere, Swiss Cheese, Parmesan.

Glossary :

Acid, acidity a description of a pleasant tang; it can be a defect if too pronounced.

Ammoniated a term describing cheeses that smell or taste of ammonia, a condition that affects the rinds of overripe cheese, primarily those with bloomy rinds such as Brie and Camembert. A hint of ammonia is not necessarily objectionable.

Annatto a yellow-orange dye extracted from the seeds of a South American plant and used to colour such cheeses as Cheddar, Momolette, Double Gloucester, Edam and many others.

Bloomy rind the white fleecy rind that develops on certain surface-ripened cheeses like Brie, Camembert, Double or Triple Creams and some Chevres. It is formed by spraying the surface of the cheese with spores of penicillium candidum while it is curing.

Characteristics, Mode of Serving and Place of Origin of the Commonly Used Cheeses

CHEESE	CHARACTERISTICS	MODE OF SERVING	PLACE OF ORIGIN
(i) Cottage	Simplest of all cheese varieties. Uncured cheese made of cow's milk. Now made commercially from pasteurised skimmed milk to which lactic acid culture is added. Cream may be added if desired.	Salads, sandwiches, appetizers, cheesecakes and as paneer in Indian curries.	Uncertain,
(ii) Cream Cheese	A soft uncured cheese made of cow's milk with cream added. The special richness an d smoothness comes from the whole milk with added cream. One of the few world cheeses made by the lactic acid rather than the rennet method of coagulating the curd. It is extremely mild in flavour.	Salads, sandwiches and appetizers.	Uncertain.
(iii) Neufchatel	A soft rennet cheese made of cow's milk. Prepared in the same way as Cream Cheese with as lightly higher moisture content and lower fat content than Cream Cheese. Sometimes flavoured with pimento and other condiments.	Same as above.	France.
(iv) Brie	Soft ripened cheese in small discs, made from cow's milk. One of the most famous and a great favourite in Europe.	Served after a meal and as a buffet cheese.	France.
(v) Camembert	Soft ripened rennet cheese, made from cow's milk. Strong flavour like that of ammonia. It is a world favourite.	Served at the end of a meal with crackers, fruit, etc.	France.

Contd...

	CHEESE	CHARACTERISTICS	MODE OF SERVING	PLACE OF ORIGIN
(vi)	Limburger	Soft, highly flavoured cheese made from cow's milk. One of the most delicate and difficult cheeses to make.	Served at the end of a meal.	Luttich, Belgium.
(vii)	Gorgonzola	Hard blue-veined cheese made of cow's milk.	Served after meals, also used for salads and b uffets.	Gorgonzloa, near Milan, Italy, France.
(viii)	Roquefort	Blue-veined, semi-hard. Has a sweet, piquant flavour. Only world-famous variety made from sheep's milk.	To be served at the end of a meal. Also used for salads and buffet serv-	England.
(ix)	Stilton	Semi-hard, blue-veined cheese. Made of cow's milk (whole with added cream) —spicy flavour. Surface rind is crinkled and brown with the interior creamy white and marbled by blue veins.	ices. Served at the end of a meal and with salads.	
(x)	Brick	Distinctly American cheese developed in Sand wiches and buffets. the mid-nineteenth century. Texture ranges from very firm to fairly soft and elastic. Flavours vary from extremely mild to sharp, depending on degree of curing.	Sandwiches and buffets.	America.
(xi)	Munster	Semi-hard, whole milk cheese. European Munster is highly flavoured and sharp. American Munster is mild in flavour, the curing time being shorter.	Sandwiches and buffets.	Munster (originally in Germany, now in france.)

Contd...

	CHEESE	CHARACTERISTICS	MODE OF SERVING	PLACE OF ORIGIN
(xii)	Cheddar	One of the most popular and well-known cheeses of the world; made from cow's milk (whole or partly defatted). Hard and smooth. The English Cheddar is one of the oldest and best known of English cheeses. It is white in colour, close in texture and clean and mellow in flavour. American Cheddar, known as American Cheese, varies in colour from white to yellow. It is factory-produced, using lactic acid as a starter, with rennet added later.	Served after meals. Used in sandwiches and in preparation of foods.	Cheddar, England.
(xiii)	Edam	Round, cannonball-shaped, bright red cheese. Produced by dipping ripened Holland. cheese in red-coloured paraffin. It is hard and rubbery in texture. In flavour it is like Cheddar, but milder and sweeter. It is made out of partly defatted cow's milk.	Served after meals of buffets.	Northern Holland.
(xiv)	Gouda	Semi-hard. It has the same flavour as Edam and is also dipped in red paraffin after ripening. It varies in size from Edam, weighing between 5-25 kg. (10-45 lbs.). Baby Goudas weighing about 500 gm. (1 1b) are now available. Goudas are made from partly defatted cow's milk.	Served after meals.	Southern Holland.
(xv)	Cheshire	One of the oldest of English cheeses made of cow's milk. A hard cheese characterized by its loose, flaky crumbly texture ad solid in rich yellow colour or in its natural white colour.	Serve after meals, or in such dishes as Welsh rare bit. fondues etc.	Cheshire County, England.

Contd...

	CHEESE	CHARACTERISTICS	MODE OF SERVING	PLACE OF ORIGIN
(xvi)	Gruyere	Hard, with gas holes, and a nut-like, salty flavour. Made of cow's milk, which is usually partly defatted.	Served after meals.	Gruyere Switzerland
(xvii)	Swiss cheese (known as Switzerland.)	One of the world's most famous cheeses. It is hard, with gas holes, and a nutlike, sweet flavour. Made from partly defatted cow's milk (known) with gas holes, and a nutlike, sweet flavour. Made from partly defatted cow's milk.	Served after meals, in sandwiches and with salads.	Emme Valley, italy. Emmenthal in Switzerland
(xviii)	Parmesan	Hard, granular texture, sharp flavour. Made of partly defatted cow's milk.	Served after meals and for flavouring foods.	Parma and Lodi. Utakt.
(xix)	Port-Salut	Semi-hard with rubbery texture and a flavour between Limbourger and Cheddar. It is made of whole slightly acid cow's milk. Oka cheese made in Canada belongs to the same family.	Served after meals	trappist Monasteries, France.
(i)	Derby	Close buttery texture with a pale honey colour. It is mild when young but develops a fuller flavour as it matures.	served after meals and for flavouring foods.	England.
(ii)	Lancashire	Crumbly texture. Has a mild flavour when young but develops a full and rather pungent flavour as it matures.	Ideal for crumbling over soups, hot-pos, or etc., Also well known for tosting quality	England.
(iii)	Wensleydale	Flaky texture with subtle flavour. Clean, mild and slightly salty. It has an after taste of honey and is pale parchment in colour.	Used in preparation of foods.	Yrokshire, England.
(iv)	Double Gloucester	Velvet texture like butter, resembles Cheddar in flavour and has a pale straw colour.	Served after meals or with fresh fruit salad and cream.	England.

Chevres the French term for goat cheeses.

Gummy a negative term used to describe an overly plastic texture, as well as overripe rinds that have become sticky or gooey. Gumminess is undesirable in any context.

Salty most cheeses have some degree of saltiness; those lacking in salt are said to be dull or flat. Pronounced saltiness is characteristic of some cheeses, but over saltiness is a defect.

Springy a descriptive term for cheese with a resilient texture that springs back when gently pressed. Ripe or nearly ripe soft-ripened varieties should be springy.

Processed Cheese : Pasteurized processed cheese is the food prepared by mixing together, with the aid of heat and the addition of a small amount of emulsifying agent (not exceeding 3% of the total weight of the finished product), one or more cheeses of the same variety or two or more varieties. The emulsifying agents commonly used are sodium phosphate and sodium citrate.

Many cheeses are available in pasteurized processed form. Among the most common ones are American Cheddar, Swiss, Brick, Limburger, etc. Processed cheeses are widely served after meals. For cooking they have several advantages. They melt smoothly and quickly without separation or stringiness. They are also uniform in flavour and texture.

Cheese Cooking : Cheese cookery is an old art. Classic favourites like fondues, Welsh rare bit, macaroni and cheese, cheese pies and cheesecakes are well known. There are countless other dishes incorporating cheese which are of more recent origin. Cheese blends happily with many other food flavours and hence is a popular ingredient.

Cheese is a protein food and like all other proteins it is toughened by high heat. All cheese dishes should be cooked at low temperatures whatever the dish is. Whenever possible cheese should be melted in a double boiler or chafing dish rather than over direct heat. Grate or chop cheese finely and dilute with some kind of starchy food such as flour, bread crumbs, macaroni, etc.

Add a small pinch of bicarbonate of soda ½ tsp to a kg. (tsp to a 1b). This softens the cheese, prevents stringiness and makes it more digestible.

Cook by moist heat whenever possible, or at least see that there is some moisture included in the dish. If and when possible, add the cheese only at the last moment after the rest of the food has been cooked. This is to prevent long cooking of cheese.

Up keep : The keeping quality of cheese varies greatly. Some of the hard varieties such as Swiss and Parmesan have a high keeping quality. Soft cheeses such as Camembert, Cream Cheese, etc. are highly perishable.

All cheeses require special care in handling once they are cut, for once cheese is cut it tends to dry rapidly. Mould may also form on any natural bulk cheese. This is in no way harmful, and can be cut off before being served without detriment to the quality of the remaining cheese.

Pasteurized processed cheese keeps well when leftover portions are rewrapped in the original paper and placed in the refrigerator. Bulk cheese or any hard cheese variety may be wrapped in wax paper, aluminium foil or plastic material. Tightly covered refrigerator dishes of plastic or glass are excellent for keeping cheese of all varieties.

All cheeses should normally be kept under refrigeration but before serving, they should be left out for a few hours. No cheese should be served chilled. The flavours of all cheeses are best when the cheese is neither cold nor over-warm.

Dishing and Garnishing : A good cook not only takes pride in preparing a dish correctly but also in presenting it properly to appeal to the different senses. This is done by suitable decoration and the way it is placed on the serving dish. One of the chief points that must be borne in mind when both dishing and garnishing is neatness. Decoration that is done without restraint or badly carried out is worse than no decoration at all. Decoration done on hot dishes must be done quickly to prevent cooling of a dish which should be served hot. The colours of the garnish and the flavour should blend with the main dish. Proper garnishing has a three-fold role in food service. It helps "dress" the plate, "style" the product and adds colour, flavour and eye appeal of its own.

Accompaniments : Accompaniments are dishes such as sauces, salads or vegetables which are used to make a dish complete. They provide variety and improve the nutritive value of the meal. What accompaniments should go with what, is usually determined by custom, based on a desire to enhance the flavour, to increase the digestibility and to improve a dish, e.g. roast beef with Yorkshire pudding, roast pork with apple sauce, roast duck with sage and onion stuffing and orange sauce, fried fish and chips with tartare sauce or tomato sauce, roast chicken with roast potatoes, buttered peas and bread sauce.

Forcemeat or stuffing are used to add flavour and piquancy to meat. They also help to increase bulk.

SAGE AND ONION STUFFING

Ingredients	***Quantity***
Onions	225 gm
Fresh bread crumbs	50 gm
Salt and Pepper	to taste
Butter	30 gm
Powdered sage or	
Fresh sage (chopped)	1 tsp

Method

1. Boil chopped onions till tender, in just enough water. 2. Add butter and star till melted. 3. Add remaining ingredients, mix well and use as required.

FORCE MEAT STUFFING

Ingredients	***Quantity***
Fresh bread crumbs	115 gm
Suet, mutton dripping or Butter	50 gm
Grated lemon	½ lime
Chopped parsley	2 tsp
Mixed herbs	½ tsp
Salt and Pepper	to taste
Egg or milk to bind	

Method

1. Mix dry ingredients. 2. Add binding. 3. Mixture should be crumbly should not be pressed heavily and not mixed too wet.

BREAD SAUCE

Ingredients	***Quantity***
Milk	300 ml
Onion	10 gm
Margarine	30 gm
Fresh bread crumbs	50 gm
Cloves	2
Mace	a pinch
Lemon rind or a strip of lemon	
Seasoning	

1. Boil the milk. Infuse the hot milk with onion, cloves, mace and lemon rind for 30 minutes. 2. Strain over fresh bread crumbs, add seasoning and margarine; stir well to a smooth consistency. 3. Stand in a warm place to thicken. Reheat and beat well; add one tablespoon cream if desired.

Sauces : Sauce is a liquid adjunct to a dish such as meat, poultry and vegetables used to moisten the food, to enhance the flavour, to provide contrast in taste or colour and sometimes to improve the digestibility (e.g. Roast pork with apple sauce); generally thickened by means of a liaison such as roux egg, blood, etc.

"A correct sauce is that wonderful production of the culinary art which forms a pleasant and exquisite accompaniment to all kinds of fish, meat, poultry, game and vegetables." The skill and knowledge of a cook is shown in no other part of culinary art so clearly and prominently as in the way the sauces are prepared. To make a perfect sauce is the height of the art of cooking.

The most simple dishes can be made appetizing by the addition of a good plain sauce while the most recherche dishes can be improved and made still more palatable by a well-made sauce. Sauces in cookery are the essence of elegance. Every sauce, whether plain or rich, must possess a decidedly distinct flavour and character. Plain sauces should be simple and pure so that they taste of the materials employed, from which they take their name. Richer sauces always require a longer and slower process for their preparation.

Sauces were hardly made use of in English cookery till the beginning of the nineteenth century. Today there are at least 650 different types of sauces and gravies. A clever cook can devise as many varieties as he needs in sauces as an artist can paint pictures.

The art of sauce-making consists in preparing liquids from various materials by cleverly extracting and combining certain flavours into the liquid. Besides this, a good palate as well as the experience and skill of the most accomplished cooks and a thorough knowledge of the taste of those for whom the dish is being prepared, are necessary.

All sauces should be smooth, glossy in appearance, definite in taste, and light in texture.

Gravy is not a sauce. It is generally the juice of meat or vegetables seasoned but not thickened like a sauce. According to textbooks on cooking, a gravy may be called a sauce but a sauce cannot be called a gravy. Many of the more elaborate sauces have gravies as their foundation ingredient. It is easier to call a thinner liquid a gravy and a thicker one a sauce.

Liaison

The various processes of thickening sauces as well as soups are called "Liaison'. There are six distinct methods known for thickening sauces:

(i) Liaison with roux.

(ii) Liaison with egg.

(iii) Liaison with butter and cream.

(iv) Liaison with kneaded butter and flour (manied).

(v) Liaison with blood.

(vi) Liaison with farinaceous products.

Roux : The most popular and the most widely used thickening is roux. Roux is a mixture of flour and butter cooked to a definite degree - white, fawn or brown colour. Flour and butter are generally used in the same proportion. Roux can be prepared beforehand and stored, but it should be kept in airtight containers.

Approximately 60 gm of roux is required for 60 ml of liquid. If the roux is used cold, the stock used can be hot or cold. If mixed hot, the liquid, which should also be hot, must be gradually added to the roux away from the fire. This is then stirred over the fire till it boils. Roux should be allowed to cool slightly before the liquid is added to prevent the formation of lumps. All roux must be stirred constantly during the process of cooking.

White Roux or Roux Blanc': This is a mixture of flour and butter cooked in a pan over a moderate fire without allowing it to get discoloured.

Blond Roux or 'Roux Blonde': This is prepared by melting a certain quantity of butter and stirring in the same quantity or a little less of flour and by cooking it over a slow fire or in the oven till it gets a fawn colour.

Brown Roux or 'Roux Brun': This is generally known as stock roux and can be prepared in bulk and stored. It is prepared more or less in the same way as 'Roux Blonde' but is cooked for a longer period to get a deeper brown colour. It is better to finish a brown roux in a slow oven so as to make it more brown without burning. This will also improve the aroma. With brown and blond roux, a mirepoix is added to give the-necessary flavouring to the sauce. Mirepoix is an essence or extract of meat and vegetables. The following ingredients are used: 225 gm bacon, 1 carrot, 1 bay leaf, 1 sprig thyme, 2 small onions, and 2 cloves garlic. Chop all ingredients and fry without browning.

Egg Liaison : This is a thickening composed of egg yolks beaten up and diluted with a small quantity of cream, milk or cold white stock. Cream is used more often than stock. When the soup or sauce is boiling it is removed to the side of the fire and a spoonful of the boiling liquid is added to the egg mixture gradually and then the whole is poured slowly into the sauce and stirred over the fire without allowing it to boil. It is passed through a tummy before it is served. This liaison is used largely for banquettes, white ragouts (usually of vegetables) and white fricassees.

Butter and Cream Liaison : Butter and cream are incorporated in sauces and soups just before they are served. After the liaison has been added the sauce or soup is stirred vigorously without reheating. The flavour of the sauce alters if butter and cream are added too soon or if the sauce is allowed to boil after the addition of the liaison. The same applies to a plain butter liaison as well. Butter is added in small amounts the moment the sauce is taken off the fire. It is then stirred with a whisk and served without being reheated.

Kneaded Butter and Flour Liaison : Knead as much flour into the butter as it will absorb, to form a soft paste. Mix in small portions into a hot thin sauce. Stir constantly till the butter melts.

Blood Liaison : This is mostly used with hare or other game. It is made by preserving the blood of hare or game to which is added a little vinegar to prevent clotting. It is then strained through a fine sieve and generally added to the sauces.

Farinaceous Liaison : Arrowroot, corn-flour, potato flour, rice flour or other farinaceous products are commonly used for thickening sauces. Dilute with a little cold milk, cold stock or water. Pour through a strainer into boiling liquid. Stir continuously until it boils. Simmer gently for 10 minutes.

4

Food Quality

The concept of hygiene is a new concept. Along with sanitation, it gives a broad based meaning. The word 'sanitation' is derived from the Latin word 'Sanus' meaning 'sound and healthy' or clean and whole. The modern interpretation of the term is broad, including knowledge of health and sanitary conditions as well as full acceptance and effective application of sanitary measures. The National Sanitation Foundation, a non-project, non-commercial organisation with headquarters in the School of Public Health at the University of Michigan, proclaims that sanitation is more than religious sanctions or a code of laws in these words:

> Sanitation is a way of life. It is the quality of living that is expressed in the clean home, the clean farm, the clean business and industry, the clean neighbourhood, the clean community. Being a way of life, it must come from within the people, it is nourished by knowledge and grows as an obligation and an ideal in human relations.

So, people need to be protected against food which has been contaminated by bacteria which are harmful. People also need to be protected against the sale of adulterated food, foods of inferior quality and false advertising. Some of these problems require government help; others depend upon individual understanding and vigilance.

Food is frequently subjected to chemical and biological contamination in a number of ways and this has a direct extensive and important bearing on public health. There is clear evidence now that a vast amount of human diseases and suffering is directly due to the consumption of infected and contaminated food.

Food hygiene means all measures necessary for ensuring the safety wholesomeness and soundness of food at all stages from its growth, production, manufacture until its final consumption.

Diseases transmitted by contaminated foods are classified as foodborne infections and intoxications. Foodborne infections are usually gastro-intestinal disturbances caused by living organisms, while intoxications are diseases caused by chemical poisons in foods. Poisons may be microbial or non-microbial in origin. Some poisons are even naturally present in foods. Deliberate adulteration of foodstuffs and the use of an ever increasing number of chemicals in agriculture, dairy: farming, storage and processing of foods is currently introducing a number of highly toxic substances into present day foods. A knowledge of the variety of toxicants found in foods due to lack of food sanitation and hygiene, faulty methods of cultivation, harvesting, transport, storage, processing, distribution and cooking, is therefore necessary for every consumer.

Qualitative Aspects

The importance of an intelligent selection of fruits and vegetables for use in the home must not be ignored. This necessitates a knowledge of the characteristics which denote good quality in the various products.

Fruits : Fruits such as apples, pears, peaches, plums and tomatoes should have full colour, a reasonable degree of firmness and an absence of surface defects such as scars and bruises.

Berries : Berries of all sorts and grapes should have full colour, should be firm and have a plump, fresh appearance. They should be dry, clean and free from foreign material, including sand and leaves.

Citrus : Citrus fruits should be well coloured and heavy for their size. They should have a fine-textured bright skin, russetting of the skin, if extensive, need not adversely affect interior quality. Grapefruit should be flat rather than pointed at the stem end. Oranges should have rough and loose skins which are characteristic of this variety of fruit.

Salad Plants : Salad plants and greens which include spinach, should be of green colour, fresh, crisp, and tender. They should be free from wilted yellow leaves. Headed types of salad plants like some varieties lettuce should be fairly firm. Carrots and other root vegetables she be firm, of good shape, clean and fresh looking. The pods of lima beans peas and all vegetables of similar type should be of a good green colour and well filled with seeds. They should be clean and bright in appearance and crisp and firm in texture. Snap beans should be of a healthy green or yellow colour according to the variety. The pods should be clean and fresh in appearance and firm, tender and crisp in texture. The enclosed beans should be small. Cauliflowers should be either white or creamy-white in colour. The head should be firm and compact, not open and loose, a condition which is indicative of growth of the flower clusters. Broccoli should be of a good dark green colour. The clusters of buds should be compact and should not show any of the purple or yellow colour of the flower. The stems should be tender, firm and crisp. Potatoes should be smooth, shallow-eyed and free from any green coloration. The colour of skin and the size and shape of this vegetable vary with variety. Onions should be dry, hard, bright and well developed.

Selection of Eggs : The shell of an egg may be either off-white or white in colour depending upon the breed of the hen producing it. But irrespective of colour, the shell of a fresh egg always has a delicate velvety appearance called "bloom" that is due to the protective mucous coating with which the shell is supplied when the egg is laid. The inner air cell of fresh egg is small. The egg contents, when broken out from the shell show an upstanding, well coloured yolk covered with a clinging layer of thick egg-white which, in turn, is surrounded by a relatively smaller amount of thin egg-white. The yolk may be either golden or light yellow in colour depending upon the amount of carotenoid pigments contained in it, and the white is practically colourless or possibly slightly opalescent. There is no odour other than that characteristic of an egg and upon being put to food use the flavour will be excellent

Meat : Good quality requirements are as follows: The flesh must be firm, the fasciculi should be small, contributing thereby a fine grain and velvety texture to the lean part of the cut. The colour of the flesh must be characteristic of the animal origin—a bright cherry-red for beef, pinkish red for lamb, and greyish pink for veal and pork. The bone must be relatively small and when cut, must be red and spongy in appearance, denoting youth; this is in contrast to white, hard and flint-like bone which denotes age. The fat must be white and firm and there must be plenty of marbling. Finally there must be a relatively small proportion of connective tissues.

Fish : Fish is a food that deteriorates quickly unless handled with great care. When buying fish from the market the purchaser should be able to recognise the characteristics that indicate freshness of the product. Some of these are: Vertebrate fish: the gills should be bright red, the eyes clean, bright and slightly bulging. The flesh should be firm and, when pressed with a finger, sufficiently elastic to spring back into place. Shell-fish: those such as lobsters and crabs should be alive when purchased, shrimps should have firm not flabby bodies, oysters, clams and the like should be alive and their shells tightly closed or if relaxed they should be closed when the fish is handled. Always the odour of fish should be fresh with no suggestion of putrefaction.

Milk : The quality of milk is determined by the grades given to it. The criteria for grading milk as laid down by the Milk Ordinance and Code are on the basis of (1) the bacterial count per given volume of the milk as determined by laboratory investigation, and (2) whether the milk comes from daily farms which meets with designated requirements.

Certified Milk is milk which conforms to the requirements of the Medical Milk Commission and is produced under the supervision of the state or local board of health. It may either be raw or pasteurised. Such milk is the highest quality of milk obtainable and is often used for infant feeding.

Grade A Raw Milk must not exceed the limit of bacterial count permitted and it must meet the highest standards of sanitary production.

Grade A Pasteurised Milk must be of similar quality with these differences: before pasteurisation the bacterial count may be higher than for raw milk of this grade; but after pasteurisation, it must be lower for grade A pasteurised than for grade A raw milk.

Grade B Milks, raw and pasteurised fall below the standards set for raw and pasteurised milk of grade A quality, but they must none the less meet specified criteria, both the limit of bacterial load and sanitary conditions of production that are permitted for raw milks of these grades.

Grade C Milks Raw and Pasteurised are products which violate the requirements for grade B products raw or pasteurised. Such milk should be used only for cookery purposes. This is especially true of the grade C raw milk.

Fats : Fats and oils may have one or more of five principal uses in the average institution food service. The uses may be as a spread on breads and toasts; flavouring or it may be an ingredient of a sauce or dressing for raw or cooked foods such as white sauce, mayonnaise, French dressing and tartar sauce. Another use is in frying, basting and other methods of cooking food. Lastly, for shortening, as in the making of doughs and batters. In each case, flavour, form and other physical and chemical characteristics, as well as food habits to which we are accustomed, influence the choice of fat and its use.

Colour, flavour, odour, consistency, keeping quality and nutritive value are important factors to keep in mind when selecting fat for the purpose of spreading or seasoning. Added to the above would be the emulsifying property and stability under heat for fats to be included in sauces and cooked foods. Oils are used in salad dressings and in browning and frying.

Fat for frying or shortening should be bland and should impart no flavour of its own to the fried food. It should resist rancidity and have a high smoking point, long frying life and low turnover or absorption by the food.

Variety of Products

These include wheat, rice and corn in their various forms. The kinds of cereal grains are the dried fruits of grasses and although the seed structure varies characteristically with each kind, there are basic similarities among all of them. The first is the likeness of the kernel to a well-wrapped sealed parcel. If the package is broken, the possibilities of rancidity increase. Early measures taken to prevent rancidity in milled products include removal of the germ in the process of refining the cereal which reduces the national nutritive value of the cereal. Regarding rice, brown rice has a higher fat content and a high nutritive value.

Food Poisoning : Bacteria enter the body through either food or water from a contaminated source and cause poisoning which, in the majority of cases, turns out to be fatal. Practices to prevent food poisoning are:

1. Observe the rules of food hygiene at every stage in the handling of food. People known to be harbouring infections should not be allowed to handle foodstuffs in the critical stages of preparation and distribution.
2. Keep perishable foods under deep-freeze or refrigeration immediately after purchase to prevent multiplication of bacteria already present. The refrigerator should be kept clean and foodstuffs must be placed in it in such a way that cold air can freely circulate around different items. This is to make sure that the foodstuffs kept in the fridge are cooled rapidly and kept cold. No spoiled food should be placed in a refrigerator.
3. Cook foods for a sufficient length of time and at temperatures high enough to destroy the bacteria. Meat should be cut into small pieces to ensure thorough penetration of heat. If required in large chunks meat should be roasted or pressure cooked.
4. Do not keep foods exposed, especially after cooking. If the food is to be consumed later, it should be promptly cooled and put in the refrigerator.
5. If the food has been refrigerated for a long time, it should be reheated before consumption.

6. Foodstuffs such as custard-filled bakery products should be reheated in an oven at 200°C for 20 to 30 minutes before consumption.
7. Keep storage, cooking and service areas clean and free from insects and rodents.

Thus, careful selection of foodstuffs and observing certain food sanitation measures prevent all the food-borne infections and other diseases which are hazardous to health.

Quality Improvement

Adulteration of Food : The practice of adulteration of foodstuffs and marketing of substandard or materials of poor quality is widely prevalent in our country. It has been roughly estimated that over 50 per cent of marketed foodstuffs available today are adulterated in one way or another. The percentage varies from region to region. It is an unpalatable fact for a nation to admit, but there is little doubt that the Indian consumer, unlike his Western counterpart, cannot take the purity of foodstuffs for granted. Despite the existence of legislation to prevent adulteration of foodstuffs, a very large number offered to the consumer today are injurious to health.

One of the causes of adulteration is that there is a wide gap between production and supply of food articles. The temptation for quick gain and easy profits amongst most merchants, slow action by the authorities, the poor enforcement of Prevention of Food Adulteration Act and leniency shown to traders in regard to the enforcement of the laws on food safety, lengthy procedural wrangles and delays, due to various loopholes in our legal system, contribute to the rampant adulteration of foodstuffs. The gullibility of the predominantly illiterate masses coupled with ignorance, apathy and indifference make for easy adulteration. In a developing country, the cost factor is the most crucial point for a large segment of the population, the cheapest product is preferred to the best. There are a large number of mushroom industries to cater to this section.

Almost all foods, milk, cereals, dais, spices, ghee, oils and beverages are adulterated. The adulterant used generally mixes well with the major food article in colour, shape, size and appearance. The more highly priced foods and those foods which are in great demand are the ones more often widely adulterated. By adulterating the foodstuffs, the merchant is benefited in many ways. First more weight is added to the commodity. Secondly, addition of colour improves the appearance of the product and hence substandard product can fetch higher price. Thirdly, new product when combined with the old one, lowers the quality and at the same time substandard commodity is sold at a higher rate. The ingenuity, imagination and initiative shown in adulteration make it difficult for an average buyer to detect it at first sight. Sometimes, it can be detected only in well-equipped laboratories. Besides the relatively harmless forms of adulteration like addition of water to milk, moisture to butter, mixing of edible oils with cheaper edible oils, many types of adulteration are positively injurious to health.

Rice and pulses are often polished with talc, a silicate containing asbestos fibre, which is not removed even after washing, cleaning and cooking. The Japanese have traced cases of stomach cancer to this practice. The other common adulterants used in cereals such as rice and wheat are clay particles, grit, soap stone and weed seeds. Most yellow pulses are adulterated either with khesari dal or by polishing with metanil yellow, a cheap soluble coal tar dye that makes the pulses deceptively brighter and cleaner looking. Metanil yellow is a highly toxic substance with accumulative tendencies, which over the years build up enough toxicity in the body to cause testicular degeneration in the male. When khesari dal is consumed continuously for a few months, it results in the development of lathyrism, a permanent paralysis of the lower limbs.

Spices, particularly because of their high cost, are the most adulterated item in food commodities. Turmeric is coated with lead chromate or metanil yellow to give a lustrous yellow colour. Black pepper is sometimes mixed with papaya berries. Foodgrains and pulses are often indiscriminately sprayed with insecticides to prevent infestation or to destroy pests; chillies are soaked in soluble coal tar dyes to give them a deeper hue, while sawdust, blackgram husk, and used tea leaves are utilised for adulterating tea dust/leaves. These are a few of the many common practices that are used today. Many cheap sweets, sherbets in variety of colours and ice fruits are adulterated with many non-permitted coal tar dyes. These undesirable colours can impair the liver and can be the cause of cancers. Similarly, lead chromate when added to turmeric powder can cause lead poisoning resulting in stiffness of limbs and paralysis. Mineral oils and other non-edible oils when mixed with edible oils can induce nausea, purging, impaired liver functions and cancer. Continuous use of mustard oil with more than 11 per cent argemone seed oil causes the disease 'epidemic dropsy' in people. Further, many mould-infested grains and oil seeds are further processed into flours and oils. Here the main danger is due to the mould growth which produces many hidden toxic substances called mycotoxins. These can cause various diseases and they act as nervous and neurotoxins impairing the general health. Some also have been found to be carcinogenic.

The menace of food adulteration exists all over the world. In developed countries, due to the implementation of food laws for the last few decades, there has been a significant improvement in the quality of food. But due to tremendous improvement in food industry and technology, various chemical substances like artificial colours, preservatives, antioxidants, emulsifiers, flavour and taste improvers are increasingly being used. Some of these pose a great threat to the health of the people. As against this, in developing countries adulteration is found to be rampant even in primary articles of food like milk, ghee, edible oils and foodgrains. Shortage of food and spiralling prices have aggravated the problem. Thus all countries in the world have to grapple in their own way with problems raised by food adulteration.

Legal Angle

In India, as early as in 1860, adulteration of food was dealt with in certain sections of the Indian Penal Code (Sec. 272,273). Later it was included under the provisions of the Municipal Act. But as a comprehensive act, it was first promulgated in Bombay State in 1899. Subsequently similar acts were enacted by other states also. In the erstwhile Travancore State an Act—The Travancore Prevention of Adulteration Act—was enacted in 1931.

Besides food adulteration, adulteration of other articles was also made an offence under this act But then acts were not comprehensive in many ways.

The punishment prescribed was not deterrent enough to prevent adulteration of food efficiently. There was no uniformity of standards prescribed for various food articles. The necessity of a comprehensive act applicable to all the states was felt. In 1938 the Central Advisory Board of Health was established. This Board in its report stressed the necessity for efficiently tackling the problem by all states. When the Constitution of India was framed the topic of prevention of adulteration of food was brought under the concurrent list and the P.F.A. Act was formulated in 1954. It was enacted on June 1,1955. After about ten years of implementation of the Act, the position was reviewed and some amendments were made in the Act in 1964 to plug loopholes and to give more protection to the honest traders. Again in 1976 some other important amendments were made to the present act to make it more effective and purposeful. These amendments came into force from April 1,1976.

Object of the Act : What the consumer wants is genuine, wholesome food, of nutritive value, free from any health hazard. He also expects that labelling must be truthful and there shall not be fraudulent claims of any kind by any statement, device or design. The interest of the trader is not only to sell the food articles to the consumers but also to make the maximum profit out of it. This conflicting interest of the consumer on the one hand and the traders on the other, lead to unhealthy practices in trade. It is to prevent such practices that the Act has been made. Though the consumer's interest is the foremost in the P.F.A. Act, that of the traders have also been accommodated reasonably as far as scientific grounds and consumers' interest permit.

Important Provisions of the Act : Food has been defined under the Act as articles other than drugs and water, which are ordinarily used as food on drink and all articles which enter into and are used in the preparation of human food. Another definition of 'primary food' has also been introduced by the amendment act of 1976. Primary foods are products of agriculture or horticulture in its natural form.

The term adulterated has been defined under Section 2 of the Act: An article of food will be deemed to be adulterated if it is not of the nature, substance or quality demanded by the purchaser and is to his prejudice or not of the nature, substance or quality which it purports to be; if an article is partly or wholly substituted by the cheaper substance; if any constituent of the article is extracted from it, if it is prepared or exposed for sale under insanitary and unhygienic surrounding; if it contains prohibited colouring matter or preservative or permitted colouring matters and preservatives in excess of the permissible limits; if it does not conform to the standards under all these conditions it will be deemed to be adulterated. There is a provision that a primary food will not be deemed to be adulterated if it does not conform to standards due to natural causes beyond the control of human agency. In short, anything which lowers the quality of a food article has been brought wider the definition of adulteration.

Counterfeit Brands

Sale of food articles without proper labelling, imitation of other food articles and coating food articles to give improved appearance are brought wider the definition 'misbranding'.

Prohibitory Section : Section 7 of the P.F.A. Act prohibits the sale of (a) any adulterated food, (b) any misbranded food, (c) any article of food for the sale of which a licence is prescribed except in accordance with the conditions of the licence, (d) any article of food and sale of which has been prohibited by the Food (Health) Authority in the interest of public health, (e) any article of food in contravention of the provision of the Act and Rules, and (f) any adulterant.

Crime and Punishment : Infringement of the provision of Section 7 is punishable under Section 16. Various offences and punishments for each have been detailed under mese sections. This section has been amended by the amendment act of 1976. Non-graded punishment, depending on the nature of the offence has been laid down. For the sale of adulterated food the minimum punishment is six month's imprisonment and a fine of rupees one thousand. If the adulterant is of such a nature as to cause death or grievous hurt when consumed by a person, the punishment is imprisonment for a term of three years which may extend to life imprisonment and a fine which shall not be less than rupees live thousand. Punishment has been prescribed for sale of misbranded food and the sale of adulterant. Preventing a Food Inspector from exercising his powers and duties under the Act, using a report of the Public Analyst of Director of Central Food Laboratory for advertising purposes, not issuing warranty, issuing false warranty, tampering of seized food articles are all punishable under the law.

Protection of the Traders : Section 7 of the Act prohibits the sale of adulterated food or any consumable article, by any person either by himself or by any person on his behalf. Prima facie it may seem that an innocent person who buys a food article from a wholesaler or manufacturer and sells it without knowing that it is adulterated is punishable under the Act. Sections 14, 14 A, 19(2) and 20A are meant to protect honest vendors of food articles. Section 14 lays down that no manufacturer, distributor or dealer of any article of food shall sell such article to any vendor unless he also gives a warranty in writing about the nature of substance and quality of such food to the vendor. Insistence of warranty at the time of sale by the manufacturer, distributor or dealer would make it easy to pin down the responsibility with the offender. The amendment of 1976 makes this easier by incorporating a provision that a cash bill can also be considered as a warranty. According to Section 14A, the vendor has to disclose to the Food Inspector the name, address and other particulars of the person from whom he purchased the food article. This helps the Food Inspector to proceed against the warrantor also. According to Section 19(2) of die Act, a vendor shall not be deemed to have committed an offence if he proves that he purchased the food article with a proper warranty, that he stored the article properly and that he sold it in the same condition in which it was purchased. Section 19(3) confers a right on the warrantor to appear in court and give evidence. The law thus protects the warrantor also against spurious warranties. When warranty is proved, the vendor can be exonerated and the warrantor can be proceeded against. As per Section 20A during the trial, when warranty is proved the court can proceed against the warrantor as though a prosecution has been launched against him.

Degree of Excellence

There are two standards set up by the government to help the manufacturers, the traders and the consumers to ensure quality. They are 'Agmark' standard and 'Indian Standards Institution mark.

Agmark Standard : The Directorate of Marketing and Inspection of the Government of India have set up this standard. This grades goods into (1) Special (Grade I), (2) Good (Grade ft), (3) Fair (Grade m) and Ordinary (Grade IV). These standards also specify the type of packaging to be used for different rent products. An Agmark certificate is issued to traders and the mark on commodities provides assurance of the quality to the consumer.

Indian Standards Institution (ISI) : The ISI mark on food is a guarantee of good quality. This institution prescribes standards for various food items and issues certificates, to traders.

Common Food Adulterants

Foodstuffs	***Common Adulterants***
Milk and milk products	Water, removal of butter and addition of refined oil.
Milk, liquid	Fat addition of skimmed milk reconstituted from skimmed milk powder.
Milk powder	Staich, dextrins.
Cream	Other fats.
Ice-cream	Non-permitted colour, artificial sweetness, other fats and gelling agents.
Butter	Other fats.
Ghee	Hydrogenated fat.
Vegetables oils and fats	
Vanaspati	Animal fat and other high melting fats.
Vegetable oil	Argemone oil, mineral oil, orthotricresyl phosphate, cheap non-edible oils.

Contd...

Foodstuffs	**Common Adulterants**
Spices and condiments	
Whole turmeric	Coating of lead chromaie or coal-tar dyes.
Turmeric powder	Coal-tar colour, yellow earth, starch or talc coloured yellow by coal-tar dye.
Curry powder	Starch coloured red by coal-tar dye.
Coriander seeds	Other seeds coloured green.
Coriander seed powder	Powdered bran or sawdust coloured green with dye.
Chilli powder	Starch coloured brown by coal-tar dyes.
Mustard	Argemone seeds.
Cumin	Artificial jeera like product.
Black pepper	Dried papaya seeds.
Asafoetida	Resins and other plant gums.
Cereals	
Wheat and rice	Stones.
Wheat flour	Tapioca flour, talc
Semolina	Tapioca semolina.

Foodstuffs	**Common Adulterants**
Pulses	
Bengal gram dal	Khesari dal (Lathynis sativus)
Red gram dal	Coloured yellow with coal-tar dye.
Bengal gram flour	Tapioca flour or starch coloured yellow with dye.
Sweetening agents and soft drinks	
Honey	Coloured canesugar syrup.
Soft drinks	Artificial sweeteners (Saccharin).

Contd...

Foodstuffs	***Common Adulterants***
Beverages	
Coffee powder	Exhausted coffee powder, roasted husk or date seed or tamarind seed powder.
Tea	Other leaves with added colour, exhausted tea leaves.
Miscellaneous	
Processed arecanut (Supari)	Other seeds or nuts broken and coloured.

Consumer Protection

For consumer protection there are a number of laboratories in central and state level. They are set up to collect samples and to analyse it. Some of the Government agencies are:

(1) Municipal Laboratories in big cities.

(2) Food and Drug Administration Laboratories of States.

(3) Central Food Testing Laboratory of the Government of India, and

(4) Laboratories of the Export Inspection Council.

Municipal Laboratories

In municipalities of big cities like Mumbai, Delhi, Chennai and Kolkata they have set up their own testing laboratories. According to the Prevention of Food Adulteration Act the Municipal analyst qualification must be scrutinised. Chemical and microbiological analysis of all kinds of foods are essential in the laboratory. Nutrient analysis like fat content of milk, contamination of water or pesticide residue in parts per million in foods etc. are some examples of the test conducted there.

These laboratories are under the Health Officer of the state. Health inspectors under him make periodical rounds of the various wards and collect samples of food suspected to be adulterated. Samples are sealed in the presence of the vendor and witness and sent to the municipal laboratory for analysis. The Health Officer can take action against the manufacturer of the food if he is found to be guilty. The manufacturer can defend himself in the court of law. Depending on the severity of crime he can be punished by a fine or imprisonment or both.

Food and Drug Administration : Some state Governments have laboratories throughout states. The Director of the Administration is empowered through his staff to collect samples which are suspected to be adulterated and have them analysed by the Health Officer of a municipality. The Food and Drug Administration has jurisdiction all over the state as compared to municipal laboratories which work only within city limits.

The Central Food Testing Laboratory : The Government of India has established a Central Food Testing Laboratory in Kolkata for carrying out analysis of all foods. These laboratories are very well equipped and carry out even sophisticated and sensitive analyses. These laboratories are the ultimate authority in determining whether a food sample is adulterated or not in cases of conflicting reports of analyses from two laboratories, the authorities concerned usually refer the case to this laboratory. Usually analysis carried out by these laboratories are accepted as the last word in analysis of food.

Export Inspection Council Laboratory : The Government of India has made it mandatory for all exporters to have their products analysed so as to ensure the quality of foods exported. Frozen food items like seafood, canned fruits and vegetables are also analysed before export. It also sees to it that ail the foods exported conform to the minimum requirements as laid down by the council. The council has laboratories in all the major parts and the samples analysed. Without the council's certificate no food can be exported.

Quality Checking Agencies

Quality Control Laboratories of Companies : Most of the companies which manufacture food products have well equipped quality control laboratories to check the quality of their products. The ingredients used for manufacturing and the products are examined physically, chemically and microbiologically. The taste, weight, volume, colour, keeping quality, packaging all these factors are checked.

In the dairy industry microbiological centre of the milk, are taken and the fat content determined, the former gives an idea of the sanitary condition under which the milk was collected, the latter whether any cream had been removed. Proper pasteurisation is also checked before supply.

In canning fruits and vegetables the fresh materials are visually inspected and all the bruised and spoiled ones removed. Oxidity of fruits like mangoes, cherries, tenderness of vegetables like green peas are determined to estimate duration of processing time, accelerated storage tests at higher temperature one conducted to ensure the keeping quality of the canned food.

In freezing, quality control checks at various stages of processing are carried out to see that the final frozen product conforms to the prescribed microbiological standards, weights after thawing and drying are taken to make sure that the customer gets the right weight. Biscuit, dairy, fruit and vegetable canning industries set up their quality.

Quality Control Laboratories of Consumer Cooperation : Apna Bazar in Mumbai, Super Bazar in Delhi, Chinthamani in Coimbatore have criteria for selection of food items which they sell in their shop. If the qualities are not fulfilled they will not accept materials.

Testing Laboratories : There are a number of private testing laboratories which carry out tests of all food materials on payment. Government has recognised certain private laboratories and certificates given by them are valid for legal purposes.

Consumer Guidance Society : A consumer guidance society has been formed in India with Bombay as its headquarters and with branches in major cities. They create consumer awareness of the various forms of adulteration and develop consumer resistance to such adulterated food products through various communications and mass media.

Food's Effects

Food is essential for human existence just like the air we breathe or the water we drink. The food that we eat is utilised in the body and the assimilated substances are used for the growth and maintenance of tissues. A living organism is the product of nutrition. The human being requires more than 45 different nutrients for its well-being.

Food materials ingested by the body are digested, absorbed and metabolised. Useful chemical substances derived from food by the body are called nutrients. A number of foodstuffs have to be selected to get all the nutrients. The health of a person depends on the type and quantity of foodstuff he chooses to make his diet For sustaining healthy and vigorous life, diet should be planned according to the principles of nutrition. Extensive research work carried out on human beings and on experimental animals throughout the world has provided us with sufficient knowledge on nutrition and health. World Health Organisation defines health as "the state of complete physical, mental and social well being and not merely the absence of disease or infirmity".

Significance of Food

Nutrition is the science of food values. It is relatively a new science which was evolved from chemistry and physiology. Nutrition is often mentioned as a branch of chemical science or biochemistry. The effect of food on our body is explained in nutrition. In other words, nutrition is defined as food at work in the body. In a broader sense nutrition is defined as the combination of process by which the living organism receives and utilises the materials necessary for the maintenance of its functions and for the growth and renewal of its components. Nutrients are defined as the constituents of food which help us to maintain our body functions, to grow and to protect our organs.

There are six major nutrients in our body. They are carbohydrates, proteins, lipids, vitamins and minerals. The human body requires 17 vitamins and 24 mineral elements for various day-to-day activities. The composition of human body is 60-62 per cent water, 17 per cent proteins, 14 per cent fat, 6 per cent minerals and 1 per cent carbohydrates. In infants the percentage of water is more as compared to an adult. In women water content is slightly lower whereas fat content is more than in men. Fat deposition in the body increases with age.

Percentage Composition of Human Body

Nutrients	*Man*	*Woman*
Water	60-62	54
Protein	17	15
Fat	14	25
Minerals	6	5
Carbohydrates	1	1

Vitamins are present in negligible amounts.

Relationships of food to health have been made from the research conducted by chemists, microbiologists, pathologists and nutritionist from the past two centuries.

Human nutrition is governed by many factors like food habits and behaviour, food beliefs, ethnic influences, geographic influences, religious and sociological factors, psychological factors, food and production, income, national and international food policies, food technology, processing, fisheries, transportation, marketing, educational status and other mass media facilities.

The benefits of good nutrition are health, happiness, efficiency and longevity.

Requisite Nutrition

When all the essential nutrients are present in a correct proportion as required by our body, it is called optimum nutrition or adequate nutrition. Optimum nutrition is required to maintain good health.

There are certain signs of good nutrition. They are height and weight for the age, clear complexion, fresh and lively skin and hair, healthy pink nails, correct posture and gait, inquisitive and alert eyes, good appetite and bowel evacuation, emotional maturity and confident deeds and pleasing personality and optimism in life and overall health.

Undernourishment : When almost all nutritions are below the requirement, the condition is known as undernourishment Under nourishment may be defined as a state of partial starvation. An undernourished person manifests symptoms of deficiencies and feels unwell. Poor body weight, poor resistance to infection, weakness, apathy and general ill-health are symptoms of undernourishment.

Malnutrition : Malnutrition is an impairment of health either from a deficiency or excess or imbalance of nutrients. Malnutrition is a condition when one or two nutrients are less or are in excess in the body. This again manifests in disorders and discomforts. Severe malnutrition in certain phases of life can do irreparable damage to the body. Physical, mental and intellectual well-being in a person is affected due to malnourishment. Emotional upset and intellectual dwarfism create personality problems in later life. Impaired functional ability and deficient structural integrity result from malnutrition. Marasmus, kwashiorkor, xerophthalmia, scurvy, rickets, osteomalacia, beri-beri, pellagra and anaemia result from the deficiencies of protein, calories, vitamin A, vitamin C, vitamin D, B-complex vitamins and minerals, respectively. Malnutrition creates lasting effect on the growth and development of a person. Permanent retardation of the central nervous system occurs due to protein calorie malnutrition in early life. Thus nutrients from food sources enable one to keep fit and maintain health. These substances include energy which gives the capacity to work, proteins which form our body muscles, bones, blood, body fluids, enzymes, hormones, antibodies, organs, skin, hair and nervous tissues. Food also supplies minerals and vitamins which protect our organs and regulate their functions and other physiological processes.

Classification of Foods : Based on these functions, foods are grouped into energy-yielding foods, body-building foods and protective foods. Nutrients which engage in these activities are known as energy-yielding nutrients, body-building nutrients and protective nutrients. Carbohydrase, fats and proteins release energy on metabolism in our body.

1 gm of carbohydrates provides - 4 kcals

1 gm of proteins provides - 4 kcals

1 gm of fat provides - 9 kcals

Cereal grains like rice, wheat, ragi and maize, roots and tubers like potato, sweet potato and tapioca are good sources of carbohydrates. Fats are considered the concentrated source of energy as they supply more than double the quantity of calories compared to carbohydrates and proteins. Though proteins yield energy, normally they are considered body-building foods. Nutrients like proteins, mineral salts like calcium, phosphorus, iron and water are body-building nutrients. Their sources are body-building foods. Just like a house is built from wood, brick, cement, sand, iron rods, nails and other materials our organs in the body are built from the substances derived from food.

Protein foods like milk, meat, fish, eggs, pulses, grams and nuts are essential to build our tissues and to form blood.

Our body functions are regulated by water, certain minerals and vitamins. They are essential for the well-being and working of the body. They are called protective foods. Foods rich in protein, minerals, vitamins and water are termed as protective foods. Water is necessary for various body processes.

Minerals like calcium help in controlling blood clotting, muscular contraction and for the efficiency of heart muscles. Iron is essential for blood formation and iodine is necessary for regulating body function through the thyroid gland.

Vitamins are essential for regulating the body process such as growth, muscular coordination of various organs and functions of several organs like eyes, ears, nose and skin.

Thus foods play a prominent role in providing physical, mental and social well-being which is otherwise known as health to the people. Health is reflected in a person's nutritional status. Nutritional status is the condition of the individual as influenced by the utilisation of the nutrients. Dietary history, physical examination and laboratory examinations reveal it

Newly-introduced Foods

Food industry has brought out some novel protein-rich foods which can be used for combating malnutrition. Some of them are from unusual food sources which were never considered as consumable by our forefathers. Leaf and grass proteins, food yeast, algae and microbial synthesis of proteins from hydrocarbons are some of the novel food sources now available.

Leaf Protein Concentrates : Proteins from fibrous materials of leaf are separated and leaf protein concentrates with 30 to 35 per cent of the original nitrogen can be extracted from leaves. Outstanding work in this field has come from Pine et al in 1961. Leaf protein concentrates can be incorporated with milk or in common flours or dal powders for children's foods.

Food Yeast : Yeast is capable of converting carbohydrate to protein. About 16 to 33 per cent of this type of conversion is possible by yeast. Thus it can be incorporated at 5 to 10 per cent level in children's foods. Food yeast is a pale yellow product. It has a characteristic nut-like taste. This can be incorporated in low cost foods for infants, it can also be used for overcoming protein malnutrition among children.

Algae : A unicellular green algae chlorella contains a protein content of about 50 to 60 per cent. This can be incorporated with soups, noodles and in baked items. Even though it is nutritionally good, its acceptability is very poor.

Microbial Synthesis of Proteins from Hydrocarbons : Certain petroleum hydrocarbons can be converted to proteins through microbial use. Its utilisation for human beings is not established even though as an animal feed it is used.

Foods after Processing

Modern technology has made many food sources into processed items. Food industry is developing in accordance with modern living. Almost all food groups are now processed into ready-made or ready for table items. Pre-cooked or half cooked items are also available. Examples of some of these items are given below.

Cereals: Starch is a polysaccharide and it is used in cookery. It is manufactured from corn, potato, sweet potato and tapioca. In the market it is available as tapioca starch, arrowroot starch and starch products like sago or custard powder where cornstarch is flavoured with vanilla and edible colour and corn syrup.

Rice is available in processed form as instant rice or quick cooking rice. It is prepared by cooking rice and dehydrating the cooked rice so as to retain a porous structure.

Puffed rice from paddy and from parboiled rice is available in the market.

Cornflakes from corn can be used as a breakfast item.

Barley is processed into barley flour and pearl barley. Malted barley is breakfast item.

Oats is available as oatflakes in processed forms.

Breakfast cereals and infant foods are often prepared from cereals. Flaked items from all cereals, puffed wheat, rice, barley and corn are available in the market. Shredded breakfast cereals like shredded wheat is a pre-cooked item.

Infant-centric Food

Most of the infant foods contain both cereals and milk and these pre-cooked cereals are eaten as gruels with water or milk. Rice noodles are popular in some of the Far East countries. Sago or sabudana is made from rice, or other cereals. Biscuits and breads are also processed cereal products.

Pulses are processed into puffed grams. Now commercial instant mixes of cereal, dal, fermented products are also available. Ready mixes of South Indian dishes like idli and dosa are prepared by using baker's yeast or baking soda and acidifying agents like citric acid.

Puffed chickpeas and peas and canned dry peas are available as processed items.

Roasted groundnut and protein isolates from soyabean or peanut can be used in the production of toned milk and protein-rich biscuits or bread. Soyabean milk powder and butter are available in the market.

Milk powders, malted milk powders, various weaning foods, ice-cream mix, cream and condensed milk, cheese, khoa-based sweets, channa or paneer-based sweets like rasogulla and sandesh are some of the processed milk products. New milk-derived products like Miltone and Chai-sathi are available, especially in North India.

Fruits are processed into fruit juices. Today even bananas and guavas are used to prepare juice. Fruit juice concentrates and fruit juice powders are made from juices along with syrups or squashes. Cordials, ketchups, sauces, jellies, jams, marmalades, artificial syrups, dried fruit and salad, preserves, candies, glaced and crystallised fruits and fruit-cereal flakes are available in the market as processed foods.

Vegetables are processed into soups, purees, canned or frozen and dehydrated forms.

Egg powder, egg albumin powder, custard or caramelised custard powder and ready-made puddings are some of the processed forms of egg available in the market.

Meat is processed into canned meat, cured meat, smoked meat, sausages, cutlets, soup powder and as dehydrated meat.

Strained baby foods with meat are being manufactured in some places.

Fish is processed into frozen, canned and dried forms. Fish protein concentrates and fishmeal and strained baby foods with fish are also available as processed items in developed countries.

All food items are processed in very many ways and they are marketed in various forms. Pickled and fermented items of innumerable sources are also available in the market.

5

Chart for Diet

Energy is defined as the capacity for doing work. From sunlight plants store energy as carbohydrate with the help of chlorophyll. Animals and men avail their energy through foods. When food is metabolised in the body, energy is released. Body requires this energy for all its activities. For all muscular activities and for the function of vital organs like heart, lungs, alimentary canal, nervous tissues and glandular tissues energy is required.

Energetic Resources

The energy requirement of a person depends on various factors. The most important factor in assessing the energy requirement is the basal metabolic rate of the person.

Basal Metabolic Rate (BMR) : This is defined as the amount of heat or energy required by the body to do the involuntary work of the body. Functions of brain, heart, liver, kidneys, lungs, secretary activities of the glands and intestinal movements are the basal activities in our body.

Factors Affecting the BMR : Basal metabolic rate of a person depends on the size, shape, composition, body weight, age and physiological condition of the person. Nutritional status and endocrine system of the body also exert their influence on basal metabolic rate of a person. Climatic condition of the surroundings also affects the basal metabolic rate.

1. *Size:* Since the heat loss in body is proportional to the skin surface, a tall and thin person has greater surface and thus higher basal metabolic rate compared to the short person. The body composition shows variations in energy use. With little fat deposition in the body the basal metabolic rate increases and thus a tall, thin person has higher rates of basal metabolism compared to a short, fat man. Constant muscular activities of an athlete demand about 5 per cent more basal metabolic rate.
2. *Sex:* Sex also makes a variation in energy requirement. The metabolic rate of women is 6-10 per cent lower than that of men.
3. *Growth Period:* During the growth period the basal metabolic rate and thus the energy requirement are increased. The highest BMR is during the first two years. After the growth period, especially after 25 years of age, there is a decline in energy requirement.
4. *Endocrine Glands:* The thyroid gland exerts influence over energy requirements. Thyroid hyperactivity will speed up basal metabolism. The pituitary gland also increases the metabolic fate if it has disturbance. Adrenaline increases the BMR.
5. *Nutritional Status:* During undernourishment the basal metabolic rate also declines to an extent of thirty per cent.
6. *Pregnancy Condition:* During pregnancy and lactation the basal metabolic rate is increased by about 5 per cent during the first and second trimester and 12 per cent during the third trimester.
7. *Sleep:* During sleep the BMR is less than in the waking state.
8. *Climate:* Climatic conditions of the environment also affect the energy requirement. If the temperature falls below 14°C the energy requirement increases.
9. *Body temperature:* Fever increases the BMR.
10. *Disease Conditions :* Diseases like typhoid fever, medullary

diseases and lymphatic leukaemia show an increase in the BMR.

11. *Physical Activities:* Physical activities half an hour before BMR measurement show high rates of BMR.

Total energy requirement of 4 person varies according to the basal metabolic rate, effect of food, activity involved, age, sex, physiological conditions and climatic conditions of the surroundings.

Energy requirements of an adult in India was reviewed by 'The Expert Group' of the FAO/WHO in terms of a reference man and reference woman. The reference man is in the age group of 20-39 years, with a weight of 55 kgs, without any disease and with a capacity to perform 8 hours of moderate activity. When not engaged in work a reference man spends 8 hours in bed and 4-6 hours in moving around or in a sitting position and 2 hours either walking or doing household activities.

In the case of a reference woman, the difference is only in her body weight that is, as against 55 kg of a man she weighs 45 kg. Instead of the physical activity of the occupation, the woman does household duties. Other conditions are the same in the case of a reference woman. The energy expenditure for man and woman is calculated considering their internal and external activities. The FAO/WHO expert group (1983) suggested some recommendations as given in Table.

Energy Allowance for Various Groups

Category	*Reference body weight*	*Activity*	*Energy allowance kcals.*
Man	55 kg	light	2400
		moderate	2800
		heavy	3900
Woman	45 kg	light	1900
		moderate	2200
		heavy	3000
	Pregnancy	2nd and 3rd trimester	+300
	Lactation	first six months	+550
		6-12 months	+400

Additional requirement of energy is needed for the growth of the foetus, placenta and maternal tissues during pregnancy. The BMR is also increased due to increased internal activities. Daily 150 kcals during the first trimester and 300 kcals during the rest of pregnancy is recommended. The energy cost during the term of pregnancy is 62,500 kcals. Additional energy requirement during lactation is for the secretion of milk. For a normal output of 850 ml of milk during the first 6 months 550 kcals/day is recommended.

During infancy the energy requirement is high. For 0-3 months 120 kcalsAg, 3-5 months 115 kcals/kg, 6-8 months 110 kcal/kg, 9-11 months 105 kcal/kg and at one year 112 kcals are recommended.

For children, the energy requirement varies according to their body weight The ideal weight of the children according to their age must be considered for assessing energy requirements. Thus in the latest recommendations, some suggestions were made as shown in Table.

Energy Allowance for Children

	Age group	*Body weight*	*Energy allowance kg. kcal.*
Children	1-3 years	12.03 kg	1220 kcal
	4-6 years	18.87 kg	1720 kcal
	7-9 years	26.37 kg	2050 kcal
Boys	10-12 years	34.30 kg	2420 kcal
	13-15 years	47.03 kg	2660 kcal
	16-18 years	56.50 kg	2820 kcal
Girls	10-12 years	36.47 kg	2260 kcal
	13-15 years	45.53 kg	2300 kcal
	16-18 years	50.00 kg	2200 kcal

Specific Dynamic Action : Energy requirement is affected by the type of food ingested. The extra heat which is produced after taking food is known as the specific dynamic action (SDA). The stimulating effect of carbohydrates, fats and protein on energy metabolism is different. Protein foods produce the highest per cent increase in energy metabolism. The SDA of protein is about 30 per cent while carbohydrates and fats exert 6 per cent and 4 per cent, respectively. The average SDA of a mixed diet is about 8-10 percent.

The activities which demand maximum energy are in the following order:

> Walking very fast, severe exercises, running, swimming, sawing wood, labourer's work, carpentry, metal and industrial work, walking slowly, laundry work, typing and ironing.

Different Levels

Energy is measured in terms of Kcalorie. A Kcalorie is defined as the amount of heat required to raise the temperature of 1 kilogramme (1 litre) of water by 1°C. But joule is the new term used to measure energy. A joule is defined as the amount of work done or heal generated by an electric current of 1 ampere acting for 1 second against a resistance of 1 ohm. This unit is very small for measuring energy in nutrition and so 1 kilojoule (KJ) or megajoule (MJ) is used for practical use.

1 Kilojoule	=	1000 joules
1 Megajoule	=	10,00,000 joules
1 Calorie	=	4.184 joules (J)
1 Kcalorie	=	4.184 Kjoules
1,000 Calories	=	4.184 Mj (Megajoules)

Energy Value of Foods : Energy value of foods is otherwise known as the caloric value of foods. To measure the caloric value of food, an apparatus known as Bomb Calorimeter is used. In this apparatus a known amount of food is burnt and the rise in temperature of water in a container is recorded. The heat liberated by 1 gramme of carbohydrate is recorded as 4.1 kcals, protein 5.6 kcals and fat 9.4 kcals.

The energy value of food is otherwise known as the fuel value of foods. This is determined by means of an instrument known as Bomb calorimeter (Fig.).

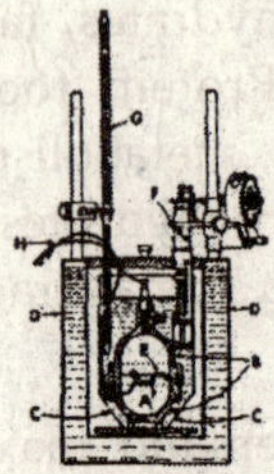

Fig. : Bomb Calorimeter

A weighed sample of dried food in pellet form is placed in a heavy steel container called a bomb. The bomb is held in place in a well insulated vessel. This is surrounded by a known volume of water.

The bomb is charged with oxygen to a pressure of about 300 pounds to the square inch. After the temperature of the water has been determined the sample is ignited by means of an electric fuse. The heat from the sample is dissipated into the water. By noting the change in the temperature of the water the energy value of the food can be calculated.

Physiological Fuel Value of Foods : Small losses occur in digestion when carbohydrates, fats and proteins are utilised by the body. Digestibility co-efficiency of western diets are available and based on these data:

the physiological fuel value of carbohydrate	4kcals
the physiological proteins	4kcals
the physiological fats	9kcals

Among these nutrients the body loses maximum energy from protein. This is due to the loss during digestion. The digestibility of various foods varies which affects the physiological fuel value.

Among the various sources of energy, foods rich in fats and dairy produce are the best Dried fruits, cereals and other starchy foods and legumes are fair sources of energy.

Determination of Energy Requirements of the Body : There are two methods generally applied for measuring the energy requirements of human body. They are direct and indirect calorimetry methods.

Direct Calorimetry : In this method the amount of heat produced by the body is measured directly. At Water-Rosa, Benedict perfected the human respiration calorimeter. To measure the heat production in an individual a specially constructed chamber, called a respiration calorimeter, is used. It is determined through the relation between energy output and oxygen consumed in a person in this calorimeter.

Respiration calorimeter consists of an airtight copper chamber insulated by wooden wall with air spaces in between. Enough provision for sitting or to lie down is made through a folding bed, chair and table. Food is provided through the opening at one end and the excreta is removed through another opening at the other end. The chamber is very well arranged for the individual to relax, read or write. It is insulated to prevent the entry and exit of heat through the walls. The chamber is ventilated by a current of air, the CO_2 and water given off are removed by soda lime and sulphuric acid respectively. For oxygen supply, a known amount of oxygen is introduced to the chamber through a gas meter with an air current. The oxygen consumption and CO_2 production are calculated using a formula. The heat produced is also measured by circulating a current of water through copper pipes and measuring the quantity of water that has been circulated through the chamber and also the difference between the temperature of the water entering and leaving the chamber.

Respiratory Quotient: Respiratory Quotient is the ratio between the volume of CO_2 given out and the volume of O_2 consumed by the human subjects.

$$\text{Respiratory Quotient (RQ)} — \frac{\text{Volume of } CO_2 \text{product}}{\text{Volume of } O_2 \text{ consumed}}$$

The RQ varies with the type of food being oxidised. When glucose is oxidised RQ is 1, for a fatty acid it is 0.7 and for protein it is 0.8. Under resting condition with no food for 12-14 hours the RQ is 0.82. In this condition carbohydrate, fats and protein present in the body are utilised.

Indirect Calorimetry : In this method oxygen consumed and carbon dioxide excreted in a given time under basal condition is measured. Many experiments on people of different ages have shown that 1 litre of oxygen is equal to 4.825 kcals when the person is in Basal Metabolic condition. The basal metabolic rate is measured by indirect calorimetry. The person has to observe certain conditions before measuring the basal metabolic rate. They are:

1. In a post-absorptive state, i.e., 12-16 hours after the last meal- preferably in the morning.
2. In a reclining state but awake.
3. Before the test the person must take one hour rest if he is engaged in any work.
4. Relaxed and free from emotional upset, excitement or fear.
5. Body temperature must be normal.
6. Room temperature must be comfortable.

In these favourable conditions the BMR is measured. For an adult man the BMR rate is 34.2-36.7 kcals/sqm/hr. and for an adult woman 30.9-35.1/kcals/sqm/hr.; for children it is more. For 7-8 year boys it is 49.1/kcals/sqm/hr. and for girls it is 45.2/kcals/sqm/hr.

The Guidelines

Planning a balanced diet within the income level needs precise knowledge about the sources of nutrients, their requirements for various groups, seasonal availability of various foodstuffs and dietary habits of the group

Blending these theoretical knowledge into a day's menu needs skill which has to be acquired through practice. There are certain basic principles which has to be observed while planning a balanced diet. As the name indicates a planned diet should be balanced. A diet is called balanced when all the nutrients required by the body are present in correct proportion. A judicious selection from the food groups will supply adequate nutrients for maintenance, repair and growth. Other factors to be considered are composition of the family and the physiological phases of family members, dietary habits of the family, food budget of the family, variety in meal patterns, appearance, texture and taste of meals, selection of food for seasons (cold and hot climate condition) and nutritional balance.

While planning a diet, the composition of the family has to be considered. Infants, children, teenagers, pregnant and lactating mothers and geriaric people need food in different amounts. There are variation in their nutritional requirements and their digestive capacity. Quality and quantity and often the preparation need certain changes. A careful planning gives provisions for all these without making great changes in the preparation pattern of foods.

Dietary habits of the family also have to be considered while meal planning. Food habits are influenced by earlier experiences in life: sensory, aesthetic, economic, geographic, social and cultural factors. Often food habits change according to the new environment, new values and availability of items. When a child is exposed to group feeding practices slight changes in likes and dislikes of foods are common. Age and sex also influence food choices. The best example is an adolescent's dietary habits. There are vegetarian, non-vegetarian, lacto-aro-vegetarian and pesco-vegetarian dietary habits (plant foods and fish but no milk, egg, meat or poultry).

Food budget is a very important factor in meal planning. Money available to buy food items, time available for food preparation, job pattern, life-style of the family members, location of residence, and family values decide how much has to be spent on food. First of all to reduce food expenditure, one must have an idea about low cost nourishing foods for selection. Intelligent selection, good marketing, just enough bulk purchase, seasonal buying, food processing and preservation, better food preparation methods, avoiding more indulgence in ready-to-eat foods, fast foods, ready-made food and hotel catering reduce food budget.

Variety in meal makes eating a pleasure. The same meal, if repeated, creates monotonous taste and reduces appetite. Variety in choice of food items, methods of preparation in colour, texture and flavour induce appetite and provide satiety value to the meal. When food is prepared in a proper form with characteristic taste and flavour, it derives satiety value.

Above all these factors, a nutritional balance in each meal is essential. Successful meal planning principles suggest that each meal must be nutritionally balanced. One-third of the total nutrients must be in the lunch, one-third in the dinner and the remaining one-third in breakfast and teatime. Skipping a meal is not good. Many people often skip breakfast which is very bad as far as the body is concerned. Studies have showed that the performance of a person after mid-morning is very poor if they skip their breakfast

Based on these principles, if a diet is planned it will be a balanced one. The Indian Council of Medical Research has suggested the amounts of various food items to make a balanced diet for various groups.

Some Clues for Different Balanced Diet —Low Cost BD : Millets, cereals, roots and tubers, pulses and leafy vegetables can be included liberally. Cheap seasonal fruits and salad vegetables lend attraction and freshness to the diets.

Balanced diets of middle income groups can include moderate amounts of protective and proteins-rich food. Milk, egg, fish and meat can be included in moderate amounts while pulses, nuts, fruits and other foods can be used in liberal amounts.

Balanced Diets for High Cost : In a high cost diet protect the foods and protein-rich foods can be included liberally. Wet surveys in India have shown that malnutrition is prevalent among high class people also. B vitamins and certain minerals are not included m enough quantities in their dietaries. Over-nutrition due to high consumption of milk, meat, fats, ghee and sweets are common.

The ultimate aim of consuming food is to maintain health. There is no single foodstuff which can contribute all the nutrients needed by the body. Only a judicious selection can provide all the nutrients in required amount. In order to select the sources of all nutrients and that also in correct proportion one must know about the basic principles of food selection. The nutritionists and food scientists all over the world have put in a lot of efforts to formulate certain guidelines in these matters. Basic food groups suitable to different countries were evolved by the nutritionists.

The US Department of Agriculture suggested a number of food group plans like the Basic-4 food group.

The Basic-7 Food Group and the Basic-11 Group Plan : The Nutrition Expert Group of L.C.M.R. (India) suggested a five-food group plan.

Based on their nutritive values foods are grouped into 11. They are: 1. Cereals and millets, 2. Pulses (legumes), 3. Nuts and oil seeds, 4. Vegetables, 5. Fruits, 6. Milk and milk products, 7. Egg, 8. Meat, fish and other fleshy foods, 9. Fats and oils, 10. Sugar and jaggery, 11. Spices and condiments.

In India this classification has great significance.

Cereals and Millets : They supply the major portion of calories (70%), more than 50 per cent of B Vitamins. In a poor vegetarian diet cereals supply more than 70 per cent of protein.

Rice and wheat are abundantly used as staple cereals in the world. In India rice is used mainly in the diet of South India, whereas wheat is the main staple in all other parts.

The major millets used are jowar, ragi and bajra. Though they are cheaper they are superior in their mineral supply and protein content Ragi is a very good source of calcium.

Pulses and legumes are fair sources of proteins and they are good sources of B vitamins, especially thiamine and riboflavin. Quantitatively their protein content is high but qualitatively they are not as superior as animal proteins. But in an Indian diet cereals and pulses supplement mutually in their amino acid content and improve the quality of protein. Pulses and legumes are comparatively cheap sources of protein. Cowgram, horsegram, soyabean, dry field beans and dried peas are some of the cheap pulses.

Nuts and oilseeds are fair sources of protein. Coconut is a good source of energy. It has also fair sources of B vitamin. Vegetables are unique in their vitamins and mineral content. Vegetables are again grouped into yellow vegetables, leafy vegetables and as other vegetables. Yellow vegetables and leafy vegetables are rich sources of vitamin 'A' (carotene), calcium, iron, folic acid, riboflavin and vitamin 'C. But the iron content in vegetables is comparatively poorly utilised by the body. Other vegetables are good sources of minerals like calcium, trace elements and vitamin 'C.

Apart from these, vegetables have a high percentage of water in them. They contribute the alkaline ash and the bulk or cellulose to the body. Beetroot, carrot and ladyfinger are high in sodium content. Fruits, especially citrus fruits, are good sources of ascorbic acid. Some starchy fruits are rich in fructose and dextrose; yellow fruits contribute carotene, the provitamin A. Fruits as a group supply water and electrolytes like potassium. Most of the fruits are rich sources of potassium and poor sources of sodium. Dates, dry raisins, grapes, peaches, lime and ripe papaya are very high in their potassium content Bananas are rich in starch content in the raw form and in sugar content in the ripe form.

Milk and milk products are the best sources of calcium and ribo-flavin and second to the meat groups in protein content. Except a iron and vitamin 'C milk is good in all other nutrients. Milk products are high in biological value and milk cream is excellent in vitamin A.

Egg has biologically very good protein. Egg white is rich in protein and egg yolk is rich in fat, iron, sodium, potassium, calcium and magnesium. Vitamins like thiamine, riboflavin, vitamins A and D are also present in egg. It plays very many roles in cookery.

Meat, fish and other flesh foods rank first in protein content. They are also good sources of phosphorous, magnesium, iron, thiamine, niacin, B 6, and B 12. The biological value of meat protein is high. Fat is present in a good quantity in it.

Fats and oils contribute mainly calories and they are good sources of essential fatty acids and vitamins A and E.

Sugar and jaggery are the common sweetening agents in our diet. They are rich sources of carbohydrate.

Spices and condiments are necessary foodstuffs used for flavouring foods. Apart from these functions some of them contribute certain nutrients. Red chillies and coriander supply carotene; green chillies vitamin 'C turmeric and tamarind iron; and garlic stimulates synthesis of certain vitamins.

Then food is classified into 11 groups for convenience in selection.

But in different countries different food group plans are followed by the nutritionists to formulate a balanced diet.

In India the nutrition expert group of ICMR suggested the five-food group plans.

They are given below:

Group	*Nutrients*
1. *Milk group*	
This consists of milk and milk products and protein-rich foods like pulses, nuts, meat, fish and egg.	This group supplies proteins, minerals and vitamins.
2. *Fruits and green leafy vegetables*	
Fruits like papaya, orange, mango, Indian gooseberry, guava and green leafy vegetables like spinach, amaranthus, drumstick leaves.	Rice sources of vitamin 'C' vitamin A (carotene), minerals and roughage.
3. *Other vegetables*	
Peas, beans, drumsticks, ladyfingers, brinjals, cucumber, bittergourd, ashgourd, plantain etc.	They are fair to good sources of minerals, vitamins and roughage and water content.
4. *Cereals, roots and tubers*	
Rice, wheat, maize, ragi corn, tapioca, potato, sweet potato, yam, colocacia etc.	Rich sources of starch, fair to good sources of proteins and B vitamins. In an Indian diet this group supplies about 75-80 per cent of calories and 50-60 per cent of proteins.

Contd...

Group	Nutrients
5. *Fats and oils and pure carbohydrate foods*	
Butter, ghee, vegetable oils, sugar, jaggery, honey, starch and egg powders, custard powders etc.	They are rich sources of energy, sential fatty acids, vitamins A and E and cholesterol.

When these food groups were suggested they were known as Basic groups. Basic-7 food group plan, Basic-4 food group plan, and Basic-11 food group plan of US Department of Agriculture was the first in these series. Basic dietary pattern and daily food guides were suggested by different nutrition boards. In India the National Institute of Nutrition of ICMR has done remarkable work in this field. Guidelines for a balanced diet, composition of balanced diet and balanced diet for different regions of India, viz., balanced diets for the eastern region, northern region, southern region and western region were suggested by the NIN and it was periodically revised based on their advanced research in this field. Guidelines for low-cost balanced diets were prepared by them for a student of nutrition. In our Indian background this has great significance.

Diet Plan

Most of us have to plan either our own or other people's diets if only to the extent of selecting from a hotel or cafe menu what they well eat.

The housewife has to plan meals for her family, the members of which may be of different ages and have very different likes and dislikes. Meals have to be planned for the school dining-room, the institutional canteen etc.

Everyone should therefore have some knowledge of the values of foods and of the factors that influence choice, recognizing that the more costly foods are not necessarily those of the highest nutritional value. Grapes, for example, contain only traces of vitamins compared with the amount present in an orange or cabbage.

During and since the war, the science of nutrition has been applied to home economics as never before and in 1952 the Ministry of Food (U.K.) published a Report on Domestic Food Consumption and Expenditure in which data are given on nutrients consumed by different sections of the community and the extent to which these satisfy nutritional needs. In 1950, the *mean* intake of the chief vitamins per head of the population was as follows:

Vitamin A	3,536 i.u. (a)
Vitamin B_1	1.51 mg.
Riboflavin	1.69 mg.
Nicotinic acid	13.0 mg.
Vitamin C	84 mg. (a)
Vitamin D	172 i.u. (a)

Including Welfare Foods : Except for vitamin D which is definitely low and riboflavin which seldom reaches the estimated needs, all these are at the level of adequacy. However, the mean figure is obtained by averaging some above and some below and that in the case of the vitamins of the B complex, all of which are near the requirement level, there must be as many individuals receiving less that this as there are consuming more.

There was not, in 1950, the marked difference between the intake of people in different income groups as was found by the pre-war survey. It has therefore been possible to make estimates of the food consumption of the whole population with regard to the supply of the principal nutrients.

Vitamin A	20.7	per cent obtained from vegetables
	17.4	per cent obtained from fats, milk and cheese
	14.5	per cent obtained from meat (incl. bacon)
	7.1	per cent obtained from eggs
Vitamin B_1	43.8	per cent obtained from bread and cereals
	22.7	per cent obtained from vegetables
	14.8	per cent obtained from meats
	12.5	per cent obtained from milk
Riboflavin	40.0	per cent obtained from milk and cheese
	17.6	per cent obtained from bread and cereals
	16.5	per cent obtained from meat

Nicotinic acid	34.8	per cent obtained from meat
	31.9	per cent obtained from bread and cereals
	20.1	per cent obtained from vegetables
Vitamin C	37.2	per cent obtained from potatoes
	33.0	per cent obtained from fruit
	10.0	per cent obtained from green vegetables
Vitamin D	36.0	per cent obtained from fats
	22.7	per cent obtained from fish

The report points out that after August 1950 when the extraction rate of national flour was lowered from 85 per cent to 81 per cent, there was a corresponding drop in vitamin B intake in all groups of the population. Since bread and cereals supply over 40 per cent of the vitamin B_1, this change was to be expected.

Average figures are no guide to individual differences. Everyone can do something, by the application of a knowledge of food values, to improve his or her own food intake and can do so without in any way becoming a food-faddist. It should be a natural habit to choose the better food when several choices are presented and such good habits can be developed easily in children.

If a mother or a school matron has enough knowledge to provide children with a nutritious diet then they are likely to grow up liking the nutritious foods to which they have become accustomed. Habits about food tastes are very pronounced and it is sometimes difficult training children (or adults) to like something new.

We would like to study various ways in which meals can be improved by various additions.

One of the simplest breakfasts taken in Great Britain is toast with butter and marmalade, accompanied by tea, but many people add to this either porridge or a cereal with milk or a cooked dish such as bacon or fish, or fruit, sometimes raw, sometimes cooked; and some take coffee in stead of tea.

The accompanying table shows the effect of a number of different additions to what is taken as a 'basal' breakfast.

The Effects of Various Additions to a 'Basal' Breakfast

Basal breakfast		*Vit. A or equiv. in carotene* i.u.	*Vit.* B_1 µg.	*Ribo-flavin* µg.	*Niacin* µg.	*Vit. C* mg.	*Vit. D* i.u.
Toast (81 percent edtraction)	2. oz	—	98	34	660	—	—
Butter	¼ oz.	284	—	—	—	—	—
Milk	1 oz.	30	13	40	—	—	4
Tea							
Sugar	—	—	—	—	—	—	—
		314	111 =.111 mg.	74 =.074 mg.	660 =.66 mg.	—	4.3
Additions							
(1) 5 oz. milk for cereal or coffee	150	65	200	—	—	1.5	
(2) Cornflakes	2 oz.	—	—	—	—	—	—
(3) Porridge	2 oz.	—	250	80	600	—	—
(4) Bemax	1 oz.	—	450	200	1,700	—	—

Contd...

Basal breakfast		*Vit. A or equiv. in carotene* i.u.	*Vit.* B_1 µg.	*Ribo-flavin* µg.	*Niacin* µg.	*Vit.* C mg.	*Vit.* D i.u.
(5) I egg	2 oz.	500	74	340	—	—	3.4
(6) 2 x 2 oz. tomatoes	4oz.	500	80	40	400	20	—
		Approx					
(7) Rasher bacon	1 oz..	—	160	125	1,200	—	
(8) Herring	6 oz.	250	—	—	6,000	—	1,500
(9) Haddock	4 oz.	70	48	300	1,500	—	—
(10) Grape-fruit pulp	2 oz.	3	20	14	100	12	—
(11) Stewed prunes	4 oz.	300-400	32	68	—	1	—

The same kind of analysis can be made of the snacks obtainable at nearly every snack bar.

Basal breakfast		*Vit. A or equiv. in carotene* i.u.	*Vit.* B_1 µg.	*Ribo-flavin* µg.	*Niacin* µg.	*Vit.* C mg.	*Vit.* D i.u.
1. *Baked beans on toast*							
Baked beans	3 oz.	70	60	30	600	—	—
Nat. bread	1 oz.			49	17	330	
Margarine	1/8 oz.	71	—	—	—	—	7
		141	109	47	930	—	7

Contd...

Basal breakfast		*Vit. A or equiv. in carotene* i.u.	*Vit.* B_1 µg.	*Ribo-flavin* µg.	*Niacin* µg.	*Vit. C* mg.	*Vit. D* i.u.
2. *Spaghetti on toast*							
Spaghetti (uncooked)	1 oz.	—	20	—	600	—	—
Nat. bread	1 oz.	—	49	17	330	—	—
Margarine	1/8 oz.	71	—	—	—	—	7
		71	69	17	930	—	7
3. *Sardines on toast*							
Sardines	2 oz.	150	20	160	1,300	—	560
Nat. bread	1 oz.	—	49	17	330	—	—
Margarine	1/8 oz	71	—	—	—	—	7
	221	69	177	1,630	—	567	
4. *Grilled tomato on toast*							
Tomatoes	3 oz.	420	60	30	300	6	—
Nat. bread	1 oz.	—	49	17	330	—	—
Margarine	1/8 oz	71	—	—	—	—	7
		491	109	47	630	6	7

Contd...

Basal breakfast		*Vit. A or equiv. in carotene* i.u.	*Vit.* B_1 µg.	*Ribo-flavin* µg.	*Niacin* µg.	*Vit.* C mg.	*Vit.* D i.u.
5. *Welsh rarebit*							
Cheese	1 oz.	369	9	140	100	—	4
Nat. bread	1 oz.	—	49	17	330	—	—
Margarine	1/8	71	—	—	—	—	7
		440	58	157	430	—	11
6. *Poached egg on toast*							
1 egg	2 oz.	500	74	340	—	—	34
Nat. bread	1 oz.	—	49	17	330	—	—
Margarine	1/8	71	—	—	—	—	7
		571	123	357	330	—	41

The value as carotene is halved to give an approximate equivalent in terms of i.u. vitamin A.

It is worth nothing that all of these (except tomatoes) are completely lacking in vitamin C, that sardines make the only appreciable vitamin D contribution and provide the only large quantity of niacin and that, except for numbers 3 and 6, not one contains as much as one-tenth of the day's requirement of vitamins of the B complex.

While these meals are useful, people consuming them regularly must remember to make up for these defects at other meals.

It is sometimes assumed that any fruit will supply vitamin C. This is erroneous as can be seen by reference to the table of fruit contents and it is worth repeating the values of a few.

One orange with about 3 oz. of edible pulp will yield 45-50 mg.

One apple with about 3 oz. of edible portion yields only 10-15 mg.

the same weight of raw cherries
grapes about } 3 mg.
pear

Fruit drinks taken with a snack lunch supply vitamin C only if they do, in fact, contain the juice of the fruit. Some brands do and it is worth examining the label on the bottle. Some drinks, e.g. Ribena and Rosena have a declared vitamin-C potency.

An attempt was made during the war years to popularize the salad lunch, based on the Oslo breakfast of Norway and this met with a measure of success although the general preference in Great Britain is still for 'meat and two veg.' However, the following example illustrates the value of the salad meal especially when it is combined with such highly protective foods as egg, cheese and one or other of the fat fish.

The value of these cold salad foods can be turned to practical use in the preparation of picnic meals and sandwiches of which a few examples cab be given.

From these examples it will be clear that certain foods are mentioned over and over again. These are the ones with a high vitamin content which should find a place in the diet of everyone.

Typical salad lunch	*Amount o.z.*	*Vit. A or equiv. in carotene i.u.*	*Vit. B_1 μg.*	*Ribo-flavin μg.*	*Niacin μg.*	*Vit. C mg.*	*Vit D i.u.*
Canned salmon	4	280	40	240	7,200	—	680
Hard-boiled egg	1	225	18	85	—	—	8.5
Cheese	1/3	123	3	47	33	—	1
Lettuce	1	363*	17	20	100	3	—
Tomato	2	140*	40	20	200	14	—
Beetroot	1	—	5	20	30	1.7	—
Wholemeal bread	2	-180	100	1,200	—	—	
Butter	¼	281	—	—	—	—	4.25
Orange	3	21*	60	30	300	48	—
Coffee (= Milk)	5	150	60	180		1	1.5
		1,583 i.u.	423 μg. = .423 mg.	742 μg. = .742 mg.	9,063 μg. = 9.063 mg.	67.7 mg.	695.25 i.u.
Proportion of day's approx. needs		½	1/3	½-½	3/4	all	all

Sandwich Fillings of Good Vitamin Content

	A	B_1	*Ribo-flavin*	*Niacin*	*C*	*D*	*E*
Grated cheese with lettuce & tomato	x		x		x		
Grated cheese with black currant jam	x		x		x		
Grated cheese with Marmite & watercress	x		x	x	x		
Grated cheese with Bemax & tomato	x	x	x	x	x	x	x
Buttered egg with parsley	x		x	x			x
Buttered egg with tomato	x	x	x		x		x
Buttered egg with lettuce & Bemax	x	x	x	x	x	x	x
Sardine with lettuce	x		x	x		x	
Salmon with tomato	x		x	x	x	x	
Ham with black currant jam.		x		x	x		
Ham with grated carrot & lettuce		x	x		x	x	

No hard and fast rules need be made about what must be included in the day's meals and what is better omitted but the examples given show how a knowledge of vitamin values can be applied to the planning of diets for a single individual or for groups of any size.

If vitamin values are forgotten it is easy to omit essentials, but the necessary information is available and no one today need eat a poor diet through ignorance. It is one function of teachers and others who have an opportunity to influence the tastes and habits of the population in dietary matters, to make sure that proper guidance is given on this subject.

The science of nutrition is a development of the present century. This has been a period during which there have been many advances in science and in medicine advances which are so closely interconnected that it is difficult to distinguish the effects of one alone.

There are, however, certain pointers indicating where nutrition has played a part.

The effect of improved diet on the heights and weights of boys at school can be compared with the increases in height and weight of London schoolboys during the half-century.

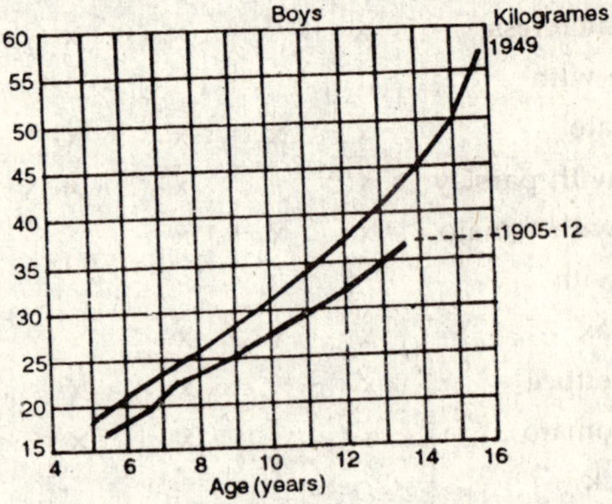

Fig. County of London. Average weights of London school children for the years 1905-12 and 1949.

Other effects known to be because of nutritional factors are the fall in the incidence of rickets and in the death rate of children from this cause.

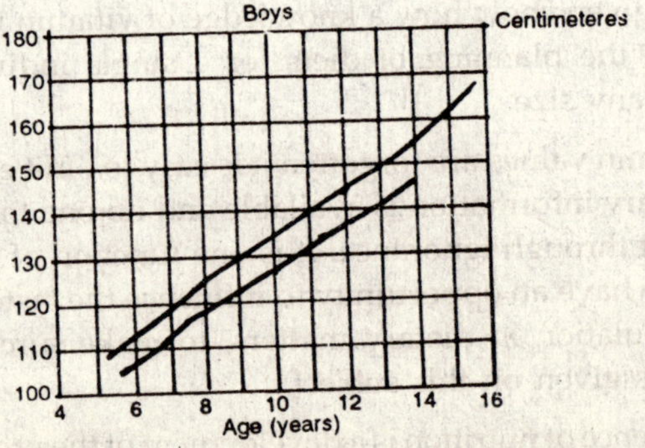

Fig. County of London. Average heights of London school children for the years 1905-12 and 1949.

Another improvement for which a better knowledge of nutrition is responsible is the reduced occurrence of complications of pregnancy, particularly the form of illness called toxaemia. Now this is partly due to improved nutrition because during 1940-42 the addition of various vitamins and minerals to the intake of over, 2, 000 pregnant women was tried out and the effects noted. It was found that the number of cases of toxaemia was reduced one-third.

The practice of giving extra vitamins has become more general and is no doubt one reason among others for the increased safety of motherhood today.

We now know something of the chemistry of vitamins, we can detect and measure their concentration with a fair degree of accuracy; some have been synthesized. We know something of their action in the body and of the effects of introducing into it, either by mouth or by injection, quantities far in excess of what could be taken in any food and this has led to the use of vitamins in massive doses in the treatment of disease. But there are still gaps in our knowledge, gaps which are gradually being filled as one discovery after another is made.

Chemists and biologists continue to work on obscure problems connected with the behaviour of vitamins. Isolated results of their works may seem sometimes to be of little importance. It is only when a result obtained in one laboratory is linked with another discovery made somewhere else that ultimately a fact of practical value to ordinary people emerges.

Such knowledge has wide applications. It influences agricultural policy, international economics, the world supply of food. These are problems too vast and complicated, but every individual can learn enough to be able to select the most nutritious food from what is available and to play a part in influencing public opinion in favour of producing and eating the foods which are best for nutrition and health.

The Proteins : In 1838, a Dutch scientist, Mulder, suggested the name 'Protein' is complex nitrogen-bearing substance in tissues. The word 'protein' is derived from the Greek work 'proieot' meaning to take the first place. Proteins play a significant role in all activities of living organisms. Due to the multiplicity of their functions the name given to them is very apt. In our skin, muscles, skeleton and in body fluids protein is present. They are essential during growth because it is the main constituent in out tissues. In a person's life the first eighteen months are very important as eighty pet cent of the brain development is over by this time. If protein is not sufficient during this time menial retardation takes place. Acute shortage of protein in early months of life brings intellectual dwarfism and it remains so for the rest of the life. That is why this nutrient is called 'protein'.

Significance : Proteins are complex organic compounds which contain carbon, hydrogen, oxygen, nitrogen, sulphur and phosphorus. Certain proteins contain iron, iodine, copper and other inorganic elements. The presence of nitrogen distinguishes protein from carbohydrate and fat. Protein contains an average of 16 per cent nitrogen.

On hydrolysis large molecules of protein give out smaller units called amino acids. Amino acids contain a drboxyl group (CuoH) and an amino group (NH.) They are otherwise known as die acidic and basic group, respectively. There are twenty-three amino acids in proteins. Amino acids are grouped into five groups based on the number of amino groups and carbosyl group in them. They are amino-monocarboxylic acids, monoamino-dicatboylic acids, dianino-moftocarboxylic acids, sulphur containing amino acids and aromatic and hetezocyclic amino acids.

1. Monoamino-monocarboxylic acid.

   eg., Glycine, Alanine, Viliae, Leuciw,

2. Monoamino-dicarboxylic acids

   eg., As paartic acid, Glutamitic acid.

3. Diamino-monocarboxylic acid

   eg., Arginine, Lysine

4. Sulphur containing amino acids

   eg., Cystine, Cysteine, Methionine

5. Aromatic and heterocyclic amino acids

   eg., Phenylalanine, Histidine, Tyrosine, Tryptophan, Proline, Hydroxyproline

A protein contains a number of amino acids. Two amino acids are linked together through peptide linkage. In this, the basic group of one amino acids combines with the carboyl or acidic group of another group of amino acids. Two amino acids are linked together to form a dipeptide and it combines with another amino acid. When a number of adds are linked together it is known as polypeptide.

Classification : Proteins are biochemically classified into three groups based on their chemical composition. They are simple proteins, conjugated proteins and derived proteins.

Simple Proteins : On hydrolysis simple proteins give nothing but only amino acids. Such proteins are called simple proteins. Examples of simple proteins ate albumins, globulins and glutelins.

Prolamins, fibrous protein, histamins and protamins.

Albumins and globulins are found within all body cells and in the blood serum. Potatoes and peanut also have globulin in them. Globulin is in haemoglobin and myoglobin.

Glutelin is present in wheat glutens, zein in corn and gliadin in wheat has prolamine.

Collagen, keratin and elastin have fibrous proteins and histones are present in thymus and in globin. Protamins is present in salmine from salmon sperm.

Conjugated Proteins : On hydrolysis conjugated proteins give a protein fraction and a non-protein fraction. In our body conjugated proteins are present in various parts. Examples of conjugated proteins are haemoglobin, nucleoprotein, glycoprotein and lecithoprotein. Nucleoproteins are present in nucleus, glycoproteins in mucin and lecithoprotein in lecithin.

Derived Proteins : Derived proteins are derived from a mother protein either through hydrolysis or digestion. On digestion derived proteins are formed. Examples of derived proteins are metaproteins, coagulated proteins, peptides and peptones.

Metaproteins are products resulting from the action of acids or alkalies.

Coagulated Proteins : By the action of heat on protein or by the action of alcohol on proteins it coagulates. Cooked egg is an example.

Peptides, Proteoses and Peptones : Peptide linkage forms peptides from amino acids. Two amino acids linkage forms dipeptide and three amino acid tripeptides. Digested proteins form peptides.

Proteoses are derived from proteins by the action of digestive enzyme pepsin and precipitated by saturating their solution with ammonium sulphate.

Proteins are again classified based on their nutritive value. From the nutritional standpoint amino acids are of two types, essential and non-essential. Essential amino acids are termed essential because the body requires them through our daily food. Non-essential amino acids are also essential to the body but the body can manufacture them from the available chemicals. Thus, the nutritional quality of a protein is based on the presence of essential amino acids in them. There are eight essential amino acids in the case of adults and ten essential amino acids in the case of children and others are non-essential amino acids.

The essential amino acids are isoleucine, leucine, lysine, methionine, phenylalanine, threonine, tryptophan and valine. For infants and children arginine and histidine are also essential.

Distance : The non-essential acids are alanine, aspartic acid, cystine, cysteine, glutamic acid, glycere, hydroxyproline, proline, serine, tyrosine, citrulline and norleucine.

Proteins *at* classified into complete proteins, partially incomplete proteins and incomplete proteins based on the presence of essential amino acids in them. The presence of amino acids helps a protein to perform all the functions of proteins in our body. A complete protein food contains all essential amino acids in proper proportion. It helps the protein to promote growth, maintenance and repair: Examples of complete protein foods are milk, egg and fish.

Partially incomplete proteins lack some essential amino acids and so they will help to maintain our body but growth is not promoted. Vegetable proteins are examples of this group.

Incomplete proteins neither help maintenance nor growth. Gelatin is an example of this type of protein.

There are certain methods to evaluate the quality of a protein. Biological value of protein and growth gain or protein efficiency ratio (PER) are the important methods used for this.

Biological Value : Biological value of protein foods depends to a great extent on their amino acid composition and they are grouped as protein of low or high biological value. The biological value of protein also depends on the digestibility of a protein food. Cooking enables the digestibility whereas overheating and frying reduces the biological value of a protein because it destroys the essential amino acid, lysine. Egg, milk, fish, poultry and meat are of high biological value whereas proteins from cereals like wheat, rice, pulses and nuts are of low biological value. Vegetable proteins are low in essential amino acid pattern, especially of lysine, tryptophan, methionine and threonine. When a mixture of proteins from different sources is consumed mutual supplementation takes place. For example, rice or wheat protein is low in lysine whereas pulse is rich in lysine and low in methionine. Rice is rich in methionine and a mutual supplementation results when rice and pulse are consumed together.

Protein Efficiency Ration (Growth Method): The ability of a protein to bring increase in weight or growth gain is considered on the efficiency of a protein or its nutritive quality. Nutritive value is expressed as growth per gram of protein consumed.

$$\text{PER} = \frac{\text{Gain in body weight (gm)}}{\text{Protein in take (gm)}}$$

Major Functions

Building Block : The most important function of protein is to supply amino acids to cells for the continuous replacement of cells throughout life. It is the most abundant organic compound in our body. It is the building block of our body. From conception to growth at various levels, foetus, infant, child, and during pregnancy and lactation period protein is very essential.

In our body, tissues are not in a static position. Degradation and resynthesis of protein and other nitrogenous compounds always take place in our cells. Tissue proteins are broken down and new substances are continually synthesised in our body. Muscles and other tissues, bones, cartilage and trabecula contain fairly high percentage of proteins. Our hair, nails and skin also contain protein. All body fluids except bile and urine have protein in them.

Regulatory Functions : Different proteins perform highly specialised regulatory function in the body. Haemoglobin, which is the chief constituent of the red blood cells, carries oxygen to the tissues. Oxyhemoglobin and their alkaline salts permit oxygen to enter into the tissues and receive carbonic acid from the cells. This process helps the removal of 92-97 per cent of all carbon dioxide from the tissues. Plasma proteins, especially albumin and globulin, play an important role in regulating osmotic pressure and water balance within the body. When plasma proteins are decreased the water balance is upset and accumulation of fluids in the body takes place. Proteins enable the blood to maintain their slight alkalinity. Proteins function as buffers, thus helping various sites of chemical reaction to maintain its pH. Nucleo proteins contain the blueprint for the synthesis, of all body proteins.

Formation of Enzymes, Hormones and other Secretions : Proteins supply raw materials for the body to synthesise enzymes like trypsin and pepsin. Hormones like insulin and thyroxine are protein in nature. Digestive juices contain protein in them. Antibodies which give resistance power to the body are protein in nature. They are known as immune proteins.

Sources of Energy : Protein is generally considered as the building material of our body. But when the diet contains insufficient carbohydrate and fat for fuel, proteins are used as a fuel by the body. Each gramme of protein yields four calories. But it is not a wise contribution because the nitrogen excretion increases along with the cost of the food.

Proteins form Part of Vital Compounds in Body : Nitrogenous compounds are present in certain substances of immunological and antigenic reactions. Examples of these are globulin of blood serum and chromatin in nucleus. Methionine, an amino acid, provides methyl groups for the formation of creatinine and choline. Tryptophan, an amino acid, is converted to niacin, a B-complex vitamin, in emergencies, Glutathione, a tripeptide of crystine, is present in small amounts in all our active tissues and this helps oxidation- reduction reactions. Histidine, an amino acid, is decarboxylised to histamine and it is a stimulator of gastric glands to secrete gastric juice. It is also used as a dialator of capillaries. Threonine, another amino acid, acts as a lipotropic agent which prevents deposition of excess fat in the liver. Proteins also help the transport of drugs by binding them into protein molecules. Contractile proteins (myocin, actin) regulates muscle contraction.

Acts as a Binding Factor : Rational binding protein, lipo proteins, transferring and serum proteins are very essential to our body for transporting many chemical substances.

Process of Digestion

There is no protein-splitting enzyme in saliva and so in salivary digestion protein is not affected. Hydrolysis of protein begins in the stomach. Pepsin, the enzyme secreted by gastric glands in the stomach, breaks down proteins into proteoses and peptones. Milk proteins are first converted to casein by a special enzyme called rennin. Casein combines with calcium to form calcium casemate. Pepsin converts this into peptones. All the peptide linkages are not broken by gastric digestion. Stronger enzymes of pancreatic and intestinal juices complete the digestion of protein into peptones. Pancreatic juice contains trypsin and chymotrypsins. They hydrolyse peptones and proteoses into polypeptides. The final breakdown of all protein fractions to amino acids is brought about by erepsin secreted by intestinal mucosa.

Amino acids are absorbed by the small intestine and they are carried to the tissues or to the liver. A small amount, that is, about eleven per cent of the total protein is absorbed by the stomach, sixty per cent by the intestine and twenty-eight per cent by the colon. The absorbed amino acids reach the tissues where then metabolism takes place.

Functioning in Metabolism : In the tissues amino acids undergo breakdown and synthesis. They are also transaminised, doaminised or decarboxylated. The anabolic activities consist of a formation of new cells or the repair and maintenance of existing ones and secretion of various substances. If there is excess of amino acids after these anabolic activities, they will be either used for energy purpose or are converted to fat

Deamination : One of the catabolic action is deamination. In deamination, the amino group is removed from an amino acid. This reduced amino group is used for the synthesis of new substances like simple amino acids or eliminated as urea. The carbon, hydrogen and oxygen may be used for carbohydrate or fat metabolism.

Transamination : The deaminated amino group may be utilised for transamination process. Transamination is a process whereby a new amino acid is formed using the deaminated amino group and another precursor. If all the amino group is not used for transamination, nitrogen freed from the amino group forms urea.

Formation of Urea : Amino acid is oxidised to ketoacids and ammonia. The ammonia, if it accumulates in the tissues, is toxic. So in the liver ammonia is converted into urea and excreted as urine. Therefore, the end product of protein metabolism is urea.

Ammonia is converted into carbamyl phosphate. This reacts with ornithine to form citrulline. Citrulline combines with aspartic acid and forms arginosuccinic acid which is converted to arginine. Arginine is hydrolysed into ornithine and urea. This ornithine again combines with carbamyl phosphate and this cycle is repeated.

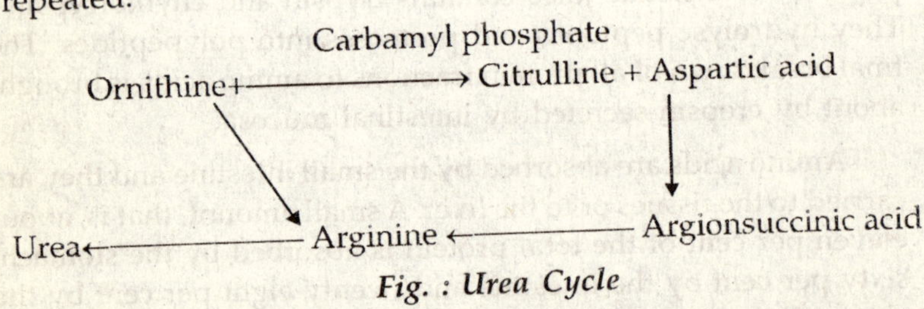

Fig. : Urea Cycle

Another catabolic change which takes place in an amino acid is decarboxylation. In this carbon dioxide splits off from carboxyl group and amines.

Nitrogen Balance : Tissue proteins are broken down at various times. When tissue proteins are utilised by the body for different functions nitrogen is excreted in urine and faeces. When protein food is taken new tissue proteins are formed. Nitrogen balance is the difference between the amount of nitrogen taken in through the diet and the sum of nitrogen and nitrogenous substances excreted from the body. When the nitrogen intake is more and the nitrogen loss is less the body is said to be in a positive nitrogen balance. When the nitrogen intake is less and nitrogen loss is more the body is said to be in a negative nitrogen balance. When the nitrogen intake equals the nitrogen lost from the body, the body is said to be in nitrogen equilibrium. During deficiency state the body shows a negative nitrogen balance.

Factors Affecting Protein Utilisation : If sufficient calories are present in the diet, protein will be effectively used for its function. Certain minerals and vitamins are essential for the proper utilisation of protein. Potassium, phosphorus, vitamin A, riboflavin, niacin and vitamin B6 are the factors which enable the utilisation of proteins. Heat treatment or processing improves the utilisation. Heat destroys inhibitors of certain enzymes and that is how it helps digestion. But if direct heat is applied to meat it retards protein utilisation. Examples of this action is roasting meat in direct heat or frying.

Requirement of Proteins : Determination of protein requirement is based upon the nitrogen expenditure pattern and the estimation of nitrogen intake. Assessing nitrogen intake or protein quality of a mixed or complex diet is difficult. Efficiency of a protein source is based on its amino acid patterns and milk and egg proteins have 100 per cent efficiency. This is used to compare the quality of other proteins.

Covering a 30 per cent addition to the variability of different proteins 1 gm of protein/kg body weight is recommended by FAO/ WHO expert group. Protein allowance during infancy and childhood is more as there is rapid growth. Studies have shown that well nourished pre-school children can attain heights and weights close to Western children. During pregnancy and lactation there is an increase in protein content. Protein requirement during various phases of life is given in table .

Protein Allowance

Man	1 gm/kg/day...55 gm (55 kg)			
Woman	1 gm/kg/day...45 gm (45 kg)			
Pregnancy	2nd, 3rd trimester 14 gin/day			
Lactation	0-6 months + 25 gm/day			
	0-3 months - 2.3 gm/kg (for milk protein)			
	3-6 months -1.8 gm/kg			
	6-9 months -1.8 gm/kg			
	0-12 months -1.5 gm/kg			
Children	1-3 years	-	1.83 gm/kg day	22 gm (12.03 kg)
	4-6 years	-	1.56 gm/kg	29 gm (18.87 kg)
	7-9 years	-	1.35 gm/kg	36 gm (26.37 kg)
Boys	10-12 years	-	1.24 gm/kg	43 gm (34.30 kg)
	13-15 years	-	1.10 gm/kg	52 gm (47.03 kg)
	16-18 years	-	0.94 gm/kg	53 gm (56.50 kg)
Girls	10-12 years	-	1.17 gm/kg	43 gm (36.47 kg)
	13-15 years	-	0.95 gm/kg	43 gm (45.53 kg)
	16-18 years	-	0.88 gm/kg	44 gm (50.00 kg)

Protein Deficiency : Deficiency of protein-predominant foods during growth period is known as kwashiorkor and protein-calorie malnutrition is known as 'marasmus'. Protein calorie malnutrition is one of the largest nutritional problems in India.

Kwashiorkor : Kwashiorkor is a term used by Ga tribe in Ghana and the meaning of this word is 'the sickness the old child gets when the next baby is born'. Dr. Cicely Williams in 1933 reported the occurrence of kwashiorkor (red baby) in poorer sections of population in Africa. Internal and external changes occur in the structure and functional efficiency of various organs in the body. Starting from hair and skin to tissues, blood, water content in the cells, blood cells, organs like liver, alimentary canal and nervous tissues are affected by protein deficiency. The child will maintain an apathetic, anaemic, anorexic, ocdematous and diarrhoeic condition.

The early symptoms of kwashiorkor include loss of weight, fatigue, reduced resistance to infection, delay in recovery from illness and retarded growth. As the protein deficiency prolongs, changes in the body take place. Discolouration of the skin, oedema with ascites, peeling of skin, cracks in the skin, angular stomatitis, cheilosis and atrophy of the tongue and- anaemia occur. Degeneration of the epithelial tissues and reduced secretions of digestive juices result in diarrhoea. Absorption of nutrients is delayed and result in general weakness and mental retardation. Liver may be palpable and soft. Fatty liver, especially in the periphery, is seen. Functions of liver are affected adversely, especially the synthesis of lipoprotein is reduced, hence fat accumulates in the liver. Deficiency of all vitamins occurs. Deficiency symptoms of B-complex vitamins lead to stomatitis and ulcers in the mouth and stomach, vitamin A deficiency leads tonight blindness and xerophthalmia, severe protein deficiency results in permanent retardation of mental development, psychomotor development and behaviour.

Marasmus : Marasmus is the result of starvation in children. Marasmus occurs when the diet is low in both calories and in protein. The term Marasmus is derived from the Greek word meaning 'to waste. Tissues are wasted and unlike kwashiorkor the body looks shrunken. The child has an emaciated look. Irritation, apathy, loss of appetite, dehydration, wasting of muscles and weight loss and incessant diarrhoea are the other symptoms of marasmus. All these result in retardation of growth and severe wasting of subcutaneous fat Deficiency of vitamins A and B complex is common in these patients.

Marasmic Kwashiorkor : This occurs when a combination of marasmus and kwashiorkor of varying degrees is present in a child. The child shows signs of both kwashiorkor and marasmus. Gastrointestinal and respiratory infection may accompany the other symptoms.

Significant Sources

The best sources of protein are animal sources like meat, fish, poultry, eggs, milk and milk products. They are otherwise known as first class proteins because they are rich in essential amino acids.

Cereal grains and legumes are the important sources of plant proteins. They are also known as second class proteins. Pulses are commonly knows as "poorman's meat" because they are comparatively cheap and fair in the nutritive content. The biological value of vegetable proteins can be improved when cereals and pulses are taken together.

Mutual Supplementation of Amino Acids : Amino acid content of the diet can be improved by supplementing one protein source with the other. In Indian diet this method has a significant role to play. For example, cereals and pulses. Lysine, the limiting amino acid in cereals, is supplemented by pulses, which is rich in it Methionine, the limiting amino acid in pulse, is supplemented by cereals. Soyabeans is also rich in lysine but deficient in methionine. A small quantity of animal foods can also do the same to vegetable proteins.

6

Diet for the Newlyborn

Next to foetal period, the infant's first year is the time of most rapid growth. Healthy child doubles his birth weight (3.2 kg) by six months. His weight becomes three times by the time the child is one year old. The normal birth length of 50 to 55 cm increases by another 23 to 25 cm during the first year. With increase in length the body proportions also change.

At birth the child has 75 per cent water and 12-15 per cent fat. By the end of one year the water content decreases to 60 per cent and fat increases to 24 per cent. Muscles would be comparatively well developed at the end of the year.

Infants have rapid heart beat rate of 120-140 per minute. At birth the haemoglobin level of a well nourished infant is 17-20 g. per 100 ml. This provides a reserve for expansion of the blood circulation and adequate oxygen-carrying capacity to the growing tissues during the first 4-6 months.

The full-term infant is able to digest protein, emulsified fats and simple carbohydrates such as lactose. Salivary secretion and gastric acidity are low in infants under three months.

Kidneys reach their full functional capacity by the end of first year. During the first few months the glomerular filtration rate is somewhat lower and therefore the excretion of high concentration of solutes is more difficult.

The increase in the number of brain cells is most rapid during foetal life and in the first 5-6 months after birth.

Diet Requirements

As growth during infancy is very rapid, dietary adaptation is required. During early infancy, much of the nutrient requirements are met by breast feeding and the RDA of an infant is based on composition of breast milk. The RDA of ICMR for infants is given in Table below

Energy : Studies reveal that basal and total energy requirements for infants are higher than adults per unit body weight. Infants require 108 kcal/ kg. body weight whereas an adult requires only 40 kcal/ kg. body weight. For one month old infant, 50 per cent energy intake is used for basal energy, 25 per cent for activity and 25 per cent for growth. Extremely active children may require upto 40 per cent energy for activity. A child who crawls or walks will not gain weight unless additional calories are supplied for proper growth. Seventy per cent of calories can be met by milk alone and rest of the calories have to be supplied by supplementary foods after six months.

Recommended Dietary Allowances for Infants

Nutrient	*Months*	
	0-6	*6-12*
Body weight kg	5.4	8.6
Energy kcal/kg	108	98
Protein g./kg	2.05	1.65
Calcium mg	500	500
Vitamin A mcg	350	350
β carotene mcg	1400	1400
Thiamine mcg./kg	55	50
Riboflavin mcg./kg	65	60
Niacin mcg/kg	710	650

Contd...

Nutrient	***Months***	
	0-6	***6-12***
Pyridoxine mg	0.1	0.4
Vitamin C mg	25	25
Folic acid mcg	25	25
Vitamin B_{12} mcg	0.2	0.2

Protein : Like calories, infants' protein requirements are higher compared to adults due to increased demands for skeletal and muscle growth. Human milk provides all the amino acids more than the required amount needed for proper growth. Protein intake of healthy infants is about 2 g/kg body weight. Histidine, which is a non-essential amino acid for adults, is necessary for growth and maintenance of an infant. The requirement for essential amino acids are affected by the amounts of protein sparing nutrients and the ratio of essential and non-essential amino acids in the diet. Human milk protein is 100 per cent utilised. Protein content of human milk is 1.1 g/100 ml or 6 per cent total energy. Protein requirement per kg body weight decreases gradually during the first 12 months as do energy requirements.

If calories and protein requirements are not met, infants suffer from protein energy malnutrition. This is a range of clinical disorder resulting in severe cases to marasmus or kwashiorkor.

Excess protein is harmful as it needs to be deaminated. Since the infant has a limited capacity to concentrate waste metabolites, such as urea, in the urine, the excretion of more wastes requires a larger volume of water. If the necessary water is not available, urea will accumulate and ironically the infant will suffer from protein oedema. Higher rate of infection is common in infants fed on cow's milk because the mechanism related to formation of antibodies to protect against infections are diverted to take care of excess milk protein. If the child is allergic to cow's milk protein, it leads to bleeding of gastric ulcer resulting in microcytic anaemia. When excess calorie intake is persistent it may lead to infantile obesity predisposing to adult obesity.

Essential Fatty Acids : Linoleic acid is the most important essential fatty acid for an infant. Infants maintained on diets adequate in all nutrients except fat, develop skin lesions and diarrhoea and growth is retarded. With supplementation of linoleic acid, symptoms disappear. Both cow's milk and mother's milk satisfy the requirements of EFA. EFA requirement of young children is 3 en% which can be satisfied by 10 g./ day visible fat. Fat also increases calorie density apart from improving palatability.

Calcium and Phosphorus : Rapid growth requires large amounts of calcium and phosphorus. Adequate prenatal nutrition supply a store of bone of minerals to prevent rickets provided post-natal care furnishes a liberal supply of calcium and phosphorus. Large percentage of calcium from breast milk is retained by the infant. Bones are poorly calcified at birth. Rapid rate of calcification of bone is needed to support the weight of body by the time the baby walks. When sufficient calcium is not supplied to the infant, his motor development is delayed. Ca:P ratio of 1.2:1 as in cow's milk is lower compared to 2:1 in human milk. High phosphorus can lead to hypocalcaemic neonatal tetany.

Iron : RDA of iron for an infant is 1 mg./kg. body weight starting from 3 months. At birth, body contains 75 mg./kg. This is about 3 times that of an adult. During the first 4 months, the baby's blood volume doubles and concentration of iron in haemoglobin falls to about half that present at birth. That is why infant doubles his birth weight by six months without depending on dietary iron. Low birth weight infant requires dietary iron earlier in life. Premature infants are susceptible to anaemia. Hypochromic anaemia can occur in infants due to (a) depletion of fetal stores (b) greater need for iron during growth and (c) inadequate dietary supply.

Zinc : High levels are present in colostrum and it promotes normal growth. Zinc is necessary for normal brain development.

Sodium : Intake of sodium by breast fed infant is less than 1/3rd that of one fed on cow's milk. This smaller amount present in human milk is considered to be adequate.

Iodine: Goitre in mothers during pregnancy leads to children born as cretins. They are mentally retarded and this condition is irreversible even after treatment.

Vitamin A : The RDA for vitamin A is 350 mcg. The amount of vitamin A content of breast milk is sufficient, provided mothers' diet is rich in vitamin A. A healthy infant has sufficient store of vitamin A in liver at birth which may last for six months. Egg yolk is supplemented in the infants' diet for vitamin A. Excess vitamin A leads to anorexia, hyper irritability and disquamation of skin.

Vitamin D : It is essential for utilization and retention of calcium and phosphorus. Neither human nor cow's milk provides enough vitamin D to prevent rickets. A good supply of vitamin D during pregnancy benefits the mother and helps satisfactory development of the infant. The vitamin D requirement of child is placed between 200-400 I.U. This requirement may be obtained in great measure in tropical countries through exposure to adequate sunlight. It is necessary to avoid large amounts of vitamin D to prevent hyper vitaminosis D.

Vitamin E : Food and Nutrition Board, has prescribed 5 I.U of vitamin E for first year. Cow's milk is a poor source of vitamin E.

Vitamin K : The newborn are susceptible to haemorrhage caused by lack of vitamin K. Breast-fed baby is more susceptible than artificially fed. Deficiency of vitamin K in children can occur if mothers have received anticoagulants. A single dose of 1 mg. of water miscible form of vitamin K immediately after birth is considered adequate to prevent haemorrhage. Excess dosage is harmful.

Vitamin B : RDA for B vitamins is based on the weight of the infant which is in reality determined on calorie consumption. B-vitamin requirements of Indian infants are not directly determined experimentally and they are computed on the basis of their calorie needs. If mothers are suffering from thiamine deficiency, there is very little thiamine content in the breast milk. The onset of infantile beri-beri is sudden in infants who are healthy. Anorexia, vomiting, breathlessness, are developed and death may occur unless treatment with thiamine is given by intramuscular injection. When antibiotics are taken by the infant the requirement for B_{12} is increased.

Vitamin C : The RDA prescribed by ICMR is 25 mg. Human milk contains twice the ascorbic acid in comparison to cow's milk though both are not good sources of vitamin C. Deficiency in mothers during pregnancy and lactation results in very little reserve of vitamin C in body. If less vitamin C is present in breast milk the infant may develop scurvy. Suddenly the body swells due to internal bleeding and the condition is fatal.

Fruit juice should be introduced in sufficient amounts in the diet from the 4th month onwards to prevent scurvy.

Nutritional Assessment : Each individual serves as his or her own control in the measurement of progress. Weight, length, head circumference, skin fold thickness and haemoglobin level can be used to assess the nutritional status. Eruption of teeth is complete by the end of first year. Healthy child has normal elimination and is active and sleeps well.

Studies conducted at National Institute of Nutrition (1985) showed that growth rate of infants upto one year is influenced to a large extent by the birth weight.

Need for Proper Diet

Breast Feeding : The word Nutrition is derived from 'nutricus' which means to 'suckle at the breast'. Breast milk is the natural food for the infant. Successful breast feeding is an important child rearing skill to be learnt and practiced.

The infant should be put to breast within half an hour after normal delivery and within four hours after caesarian operational birth cases. Prelacteral foods like honey, distilled water or glucose should not be given. These foods will satisfy the thirst and will reduce the vigour to suck and may lead to diarrhoea and helminthic infestation. Breast feeding can be initiated even when the mother is sedated or on IV fluids.

Colostrum : During the first two or three days watery and yellowish fluid that comes from the mammary gland differs from the regular milk and is called colostrum. It is secreted in small quantity of about 10-40 ml. It is rich in protein. The total fat content of colostrum is less than mature milk. The concentration of lactose is also less. The levels of niacin, pantothenic acid, biotin and riboflavin are also low. Vitamin C is secreted at about the same level as in mature milk. Zinc content of colostrum is 20 mg/1. whereas mature milk has 2.6 mg/1. The composition of colostrum is given in the Table below.

Composition of Colostrum

Nutrient	*Amount*
Energy kcal	58
Fat g	2.9
Calcium mg	31
Phosphorus mg	14
Iron mg	0.09
Protein g	2.7
Lactose g	5.3
Carotene I.U	186
Vitamin A.I.U	296

Colostrum contains an interferon like substance which possesses strong antiviral activity. Colostrum contains B_{12} binding protein which renders B_{12} unavailable for the growth of E. Coli and other bacteria. It also contains antibodies against viral diseases such as small pox, polio, measles and influenza. Enzymes like lysozyme, peroxidase and xanthine oxidase that promote cell maturation are found to be more in colostrum.

Advantages of Breast Feeding : Any woman who delivers a child can breast feed the off spring. Breast feeding is not only beneficial to the infant but also to the mother. The advantages of breast feeding can be considered under nutritional, immunological, psychological, economical and physiological and other factors.

Nutritional Factors : The composition of human milk is best suited to the infants. The table below shows the comparative data of human milk with cow's and buffalo's milk.

Comparison of Human Milk with Cow's and Buffalo's Milk

Nutrient	*Human milk*	*Cow's milk (Values per 100 g.)*	*Buffalo's milk*
Water g	88	87.5	81
Energy kcal	65	67	117
Protein g	1.1	3.2	4.3
Carbohydrate g	7.4	4.4	5
Fat g	3.4	4.1	6.5
Calcium mg	28	120	210
Phosphorus mg	11	90	130
Iron mg	—	0.2	0.2
Carotene mcg	137	174	160
Thiamine mg	0.02	0.05	0.04
Riboflavin mg	0.02	0.19	0.1
Vitamin C mg	3	2	1
Caseinogen and Lactalbumin ratio	1:2	3:1	—

Energy : Calorie value of human milk and cow's milk are similar as is the total fat content. Lower protein content of human milk is compensated by higher amount of lactose. Table below shows the percentage calories from protein, fat and carbohydrate in human and cow's milk.

Calories percentage from Protein, Fat and Carbohydrate in Human and Cow's Milk

Nutrient	*Human milk*	*Cow's milk*
Total energy (per 100 ml)	65	67
Protein	7	19
Fat	47	55
Carbohydrates	31	26

From the above table it is clear that human milk protein calorie per cent is less than cow's milk whereas carbohydrate calorie per cent is higher in human milk. Ideally for an infant 6 per cent of calories should come from protein. Fat content in human milk is comparatively less. It is advantageous, as it is absorbed easily.

In first 24 hours, glycogen is used for energy. Later on glucose and fatty acid from the diet or from body fat stores are used up. Free fatty acids are released from triglycerides by lipase which is present in human milk. These are preferred source of energy for the infants heart, throughout the sucking period. The switch over to fatty acid calls for a source of carnitine to transport fatty acid within the cell. Newborns do not have a fully developed ability to synthesise carnitine and they must obtain it from breast milk or from formulas where carnitine is added. Carnitine is absent in cow's milk.

Carbohydrate : Human milk is the sweetest milk due to the high amount of lactose. Lactose which is present in higher levels in human milk facilitates the absorption of magnesium and calcium and favours amino acid absorption and nitrogen retention. Galactose is present only in milk and is essential for the formation of myelin, which in turn is essential for the normal nerve function. (Myelin is a protective sheath that surrounds the nerve fibre and protects their ability to transmit nerve messages.) High content of galacto lipids promote rapid brain growth of infant. Lactose which is least soluble cannot be added to milk at home. Lactose is added in commercial formulas. Sucrose if added may cause gastrointestinal distress in infants. Human milk contains a salivary enzyme-like amylase which helps in digesting starch at a stage in life when little or no pancreatic amylase is produced.

Protein : Human milk contains 1.1g % protein. The protein content in cow's milk is three times more than that in human milk. However it is biochemically different and less digestible.

Human milk has 20% beta-casein and 80% whey proteins which constitute lactalbumin and lactoferrin. Cow's milk has 80% alpha-casein and 20% whey proteins which constitute lactoglobulin. This lactoglobulin is one of the causes of intolerance to cow's milk. Beta lactoglobulin which is an allergen is absent in human milk.

Lactalbumin has an amino acid pattern that mainly approaches that of body protein and provides more essential amino acids than does casein. Among the amino acids, glutamic acid is maximum and glycine is absent in human milk.

Casein forms a hard curd with rennin and lactalbumin forms a soft flocculent curd that is most rapidly digested and absorbed by the infant.

Human milk with its low protein and solute load is suitable for the slower somatic growth in the baby for rapid brain growth in the first year of life. Breast milk contains amino acids specific for brain development. It is rich in sulphur containing amino aids, cysteine, methionine ratio is high and this compensates for low cysteine methionine conversion which is essential for central nervous system development. Taurine is an important neuro-transmitter and neuro-modulator for brain and retina. Taurine is present in large amounts in human milk than in cow's milk.

Human milk offers a high tryptophan to neutral amino acids ratio which controls brain serotonin synthesis.

Human milk also contains binding proteins of thyroxine, corticosterol, vitamin D, folate and $B_{12.}$

Even though protein content is low in human milk, non-protein nitrogen are high and net nitrogen content is comparable in human and cow's milk. The non-protein nitrogens in human milk are urea, amino acids, peptides, nucleic acids, N-acetyl glutamine and N- acetyl neuraminic acid.

Presence of protein splitting enzymes in breast milk reduces protein to the less complex peptone stage, on which digestive enzymes act more effectively. These enzymes in cow's milk are destroyed by the heat of pasteurisation.

Lipids : Lipids present in human milk, are unsaturated fat, essential fatty acids, prostaglandin precursors, fat soluble vitamins, steroids, phospholipid and cholesterol.

Infants have only a limited ability to convert alpha-linolenic acid to eicosa pentaenoic acid (EPA) and docosa hexaenoic acid (DHA) but these are present in human milk. In cow's milk and infant formula on the other hand, EPA and DHA are either absent or present at low levels.

Brain lipids are mostly long chain polyunsaturated fatty acids which are abundant in breast milk. DHA is important for neural division. If mother's intake of fish is increased the level of EPA and DHA in milk can be increased. Type of fat present in human milk depends on dietary fat of the mother.

Human milk also has high carnitine content which increases metabolism by mitochondrial oxidation and transport of essential fatty acid. Human milk contains cholesterol and is essential for the synthesis of myelin of the nervous system. Presence of choline, acetylcholine, phospholipid precursors and carnitine ensure optimum metabolism and brain development.

Breast milk, meets the essential fatty acid needs of infants which is about 6 en% . The polyunsaturated to saturated fat ratio is 1.2 : 1 in breast milk, compared to 1:2 in cow's milk.

The increase in the fat content of human milk from the beginning of feeding to the end is believed to increase its satiety value and to make it easier for the breast-fed infant to regulate caloric intake and weight gain.

Minerals : Unlike vitamins, mineral content of human milk is minimally influenced by the mother's stores and immediate intake of calcium, magnesium, phosphorus, iron, copper, zinc, sodium and potassium.

Calcium content in human milk is 28 mg and in cow's milk 120 mg. Though the calcium content of human milk is 1/4th of cow's milk, calcium phosphorus ratio of 2:1 in human milk is favourable. Infantile tetany rarely occurs in breast-fed infants.

Low sodium content of human milk is advantageous to the infant as kidneys have difficulty in handling excess sodium. Sodium content of milk, is influenced by diet.

Though iron content is low in human milk a full-term infant

needs only 0.3 mg/day and human milk meets this requirement. Iron is more available, in the presence of lactoferrin in human milk. Human milk enhances zinc absorption. Human milk has high Cu: Zn ratio 1:5 and cow's milk has 1:15 ratio. Copper content of human milk is more. No copper deficiency is found in breast-fed infants.

Breast milk ensures better oxygen saturation and increases the bio-availability of trace elements like copper, cobalt, selenium, iron and zinc.

It contains less poisonous residues than cow's milk which are neurotoxic like chromium, aluminum and manganese.

Vitamins : The vitamin content of human milk generally reflects the vitamin intake and nutritional status of the mother.

Breast milk contains more vitamin A, C and E than cow's milk. Xerophthalmia and Keratomalacia can occur in the first year of life among artificially fed infants but rare among breast fed. Breast milk contains water soluble vitamin D along with fat soluble fraction which protects against rickets. Vitamin D content of human milk reflects maternal intakes and nutritional status of the mother. Human milk may be low in vitamin K and all infants should receive vitamin K supplement soon after birth.

Riboflavin, pyridoxine and B_{12} content of human milk are also related to the dietary intake of mother. Heat labile vitamins like thiamine and ascorbic acid, are completely available in human milk. Cow's milk is heated before consumption and these heat labile vitamins may be lost.

Breast-fed infants receive about 25-30 μg of folate daily, most of which is available for absorption.

Hormones and Growth Factors : Breast milk is a rich source of hormones like thyroid stimulating hormone (TSH), thyroxine, growth hormone releasing factor, insulin and prolactin. It contains growth regulating factors, growth promoting factors and growth modulators.

Immunological Factors : These factors are present in colostrum as well as in matured milk. Colostrum particles which have anti-infective properties of human milk are stable in acid medium of the stomach and resistant to the digestive enzymes.

With different factors bestow passive immunity, that is, they provide a form of immunity that does not require the activation of the infant's own immune defenses.

Macrophages : They contribute immunity in two ways:

a. They engulf and digest bacteria.
b. These cells synthesize complement, a protein involved in establishing immunity to infectious organism.

The bacteria and viruses that are responsible for diseases such as poliomyelitis, influenza and diptheria can be destroyed by this way.

Lymphocytes : Lymphocytes are the white blood cells responsible for mediating most aspects of the immune system, with its ability to attack a wide range of infectious microorganisms. Human milk contains T and B lymphocytes. T. lymphocytes are responsible for transfer of immunological memory. Transfer of maternal antibodies and T. lymphocytes may offer some protection against malaria.

Lymphocytes produce lymphokynes and other growth factors which stimulate proliferation and differentiation in lymphoid tissue and its capacity to react antigens. Lymphocytes also produce an antiviral substance called interferon.

These cells in breast milk may therefore play an important role in the infant's transition from passive to active immunity.

Lactoferrin : It is an iron containing protein found both in colostrum and mature milk. It inhibits the growth of staphylococcus organism and E. Coli by tying of the iron they need for growth. By removing free iron and thus preventing bacterial proliferation and free radical generation, lactoferrin has a protective effect. If excess of iron is provided in the diet the infant is susceptible for infection.

Lactobacillus Bifidus Factor : The bifidus factor as Gyorgy called it, is present in human milk in a concentration 40 times greater than in cow's milk. It is an amino sugar and contains

N-acetyl neuraminic acid, a substance that has a very wide biological role.

It is a nitrogen containing carbohydrate in human milk. It encourages the growth of microorganism, lactobacillus bifidus and produces acetic acid or lactic acid from lactose and depresses the growth of pathogenic or disease producing organisms like Escherichia coli. Growth of lactobacillus bifidus is enhanced on a high lactose and low protein diet. Lactose/protein ratio in human milk is 7:1 compared to cow's milk which is 4:1.

Enzymes : Breast milk supplies enzymes like amylase, lipoprotein lipase, bile salt stimulated lipases, oxidases, lacto peroxidase and leucocyte myeloperioxidase. These enzymes increase digestibility and also act as defence against microbes. Lipases kill bacteria. Bile salt stimulated lipase kills amoeba and giardia. Lysozyme digests the cell wall of bacteria after the bacteria have been inactivated by the peroxide and vitamin C. Lactoperoxidase attacks the streptococcus organism.

Enzymes like lysozyme, peroxidase and xanthine oxidase promote cell maturation.

Immunoglobulins : Immunoglobulins are the defensive proteins that include all types of antibodies. Secretary IgA plays a major role in defending an infant against viruses, bacteria and other pathogens and harmful food components in the first few days of life. It acts within the gastrointestinal tract and is especially effective against pathogens to which the mother has been exposed such as polio virus, streptococcus and pneumococcus.

Human milk also contains IgG and IgM immunoglobulins but at a much lower level than that of IgA. It is interesting that the infant makes relatively low levels of its own IgA immunoglobulin and high levels of its own IgG and IgM immunoglobulin during the first year of life. This is an example of the functional development of the infant working in harmony with the composition of the milk it receives from its mother. Immunoglobulin are resistant to the acidity of the stomach.

Research indicates that breast feeding must be maintained

until the infant is at least 3 months of age in order for this protection to be conferred.

Fatty Acids and Monoglycerides : These are present in human milk and are able to penetrate the membranes of viruses and bacteria and destroy them. They contribute for passive immunity and provide protection without the use of medicines or vaccines.

Para Amino Benzoic Acid : Para Amino Benzoic Acid is absolutely essential for erythrocytic stages of malarial parasite. Lack of PABA in human milk inhibits malaria.

Human milk may be useful in the treatment of protracted diarrhoea presumably through local effects in the gut. More generally, the ability of the mother to secrete antibodies directed against specific antigens in her environment, imparts to human milk an environmental specificity with significant protective potential.

Breast feeding is associated with reduced need for hospitalisation and improved child survival.

Psychological Factors : An infant derives a sense of security and belonging in the mother and child relationship from the comfort of being held than from feeding process. Mother also feels that she is involved in a unique process for which there is no substitute.

Economic Factors : It is economical to breast-feed an infant, even though mother's requirements are increased. Commercial preparations are expensive. In artificial feeding money has to be spent not only for the milk or milk powder but for sterilising the equipment also. Also there is no wastage of human milk.

Immunological Factors in Human Milk

* Immunoglobins : Secretory IgA, IgG, IgM
* Cellular elements : Lymphoid cells, polymorphs, macrophages, plasma cells.
* Opsonic and chemotactic activities of C_3 and C_4 complement system.
* Unsaturated lactoferin and transferrin.
* Lysozyme
* Lactoperoxidase

* Specific inhibitors (non-immunoglobulins) antiviral and anti-staphylococcal factors.
* Growth factors for lactobacillus bifidus.
* Para-amino benzoic acid may afford some protection against malaria.

Physiological Factors : Breast-feeding is an important birth control method. Prolactin which stimulates milk production, decreases the synthesis of ovarian hormones. It is the most cost effective method of family planning.

When the mother feeds the infant, the uterus comes back to normal size and arrests bleeding due to the secretion of oxytocin. Breast-feeding enables the mother to shed extra weight accumulated during pregnancy under the effect of various hormones.

Other Factors

a. Infants' jaw is more fully developed and teeth are less crowded as he works harder to extract milk.
b. Micobiologically it is sterile and less danger of contamination and gastro-intestinal problems. Mortality rate is lower in children who are breast-fed.
c. Low danger of incorrect formula and overfeeding.
d. Reduced chances of allergic reactions, as human milk protein do not cause allergies.
e. Lower rate of sudden infant death or cot death. As infant will not be sensitive to human milk and less possibility of aspiration following regurgitation or higher vitamin E in human milk will protect the membrane in the lungs.
f. Less renal solute load as there is less urea and sodium to excrete.
g. Less colic as fats and protein in human milk are more easily digested and less likely to create gastric and intestinal distress.
h. Human milk is always fresh and at the right temperature. It has optimum fluidity,
i. It is convenient to administer for the mother at any place and time.

j. Breast feeding can be continued during illness of the infant, like diarrhoea.

k. Risk of breast cancer is higher in women who have not breast-fed their children.

l. There is evidence to suggest that breast-fed babies are less likely to develop obesity, hypertension, diabetes mellitus and atherosclerosis in later life. Late onset tetany, metabolic acidosis and acrodermatitis enteropathica are limited to top fed babies.

m. There is evidence to suggest that breast fed babies have better cognition and IQ score later in life.

n. It is one food that makes a complete meal. Meal is always ready, no preparation and no left overs.

o. Breast milk is a renewable resource. It cannot be adulterated. Breast feeding can be continued during most of the maternal illnesses including mastitis, breast abscess, TB and hepatitis B. Breast feeding can be given during infections, rhinitis, viral fever, respiratory infections, asthma etc. It should be discontinued only if there are gastrointestinal contra indications to oral feedings. Breast feeding can be continued by the poor mother as long as she is able to feed but supplementary feeding should be started from 6th month onwards.

Recommendations for Promotion of Successful Breast Feeding

- Education and advice must be given to every mother in the antenatal clinic. Retracted and crackled nipples must be managed before delivery.
- The first feed should be breast milk (no water, honey, glucose water tea etc. should be given).
- Breast feeding should preferably be started in the first hour of life.
- Bottle feeds should never be introduced.
- A breast feed baby does not require supplementation with water.

- Frequent suckling, complete emptying of the breast, correct positioning and supportive care are the corner stones of successful lactation.

Realising that aggressive marketing of infant foods and feeding bottles leads to a decline in breast-feeding, the World Health Assembly in 1981 passed an International code of Marketing of Breast milk substitutes. In 1992, the government of India passed the Infant Milk Substitutes, feeding bottles and Infant Foods Act 1992, which came into force 1st August 1993.

Infant Milk Substitute (IMS) Act 1992 : The IMS, feeding bottles and infant foods (Regulation, production, supply and distribution) Act 1992 was passed to protect, promote and support breast feeding. The salient features of the act are the following.

- There should be no promotion of infant feeding products in health care facilities.
- Booklets, leaflets, brochures, posters, feeding bottles, cot tags, stickers, clinic cards, prescription pads and similar materials which advertise infant feeding products should not be permitted.
- There should be no display of artificial infant feeding products in health care facilities.
- Company marketing personnel, no matter what they are called, should not be permitted to have contact with mothers.
- Artificial infant feeding should be the exception and not the rule. Only parents who need to artificially feed their infants should be instructed. Instruction should be given only by health or community workers. The instructions should include a clear warning about the health hazards of artificial feeding.

Breast milk is not only the best but it is a must for the infant.

UNICEF and WHO have initiated a scheme called "The Baby friendly Hospital Initiative" to impart health education which includes breast feeding to rural women who deliver at home and who are unaware of the modern health care system.

World Alliance for Breast feeding Action (WABA) has designated August 1-7 as the world breast feeding week. WABA is a network of organisations and individuals in collaboration with the WHO and UNICEF to protect, promote and support breast feeding as natural and inherent right of all newborn babies and mothers.

Understanding the importance of it, "breast milk bank" is in operation at KEM Hospital, Mumbai for infants who cannot get their mother's milk.

Factors like lack of suitable information, inappropriate health practices, biased health professionals and aggressive promotion of milk substitutes discourage breast feeding.

According to Breast feeding Promotion Network of India (BPNI) studies there was a decline in breast feeding during the last decade, especially during first four months of life.

Support from Outside

Though no milk can be a real substitute for mother's milk, sometimes it is needed to give artificial feeding. Circumstances under which artificial feeding is essential are:

(1) The mother is suffering from serious illness, fever or infection.

(2) Another pregnancy intervenes during lactation.

(3) The child is too weak to nurse or cannot because of harelip or cleft palate.

(4) Breast milk has completely stopped or insufficient for the child.

(5) Mother is not available to feed the child.

(6) The mother is on anticoagulants, steroids and radioactive drugs.

(7) Death of the mother.

Advantages of Bottle Feeding

- Creates no additional requirements in the mother.
- No problems in establishing the milk supply.
- The volume of milk given is visible.

- Feeding in public is acceptable.
- Less jealousy may be incurred because other members of the family can feed the baby.
- Creates no problems for the working mother.
- Provided the correct amount is given it will be nutritionally adequate.

Modification of the Formula : Cow's milk is diluted to provide a concentration of protein similar to that of human milk. And also this leads to the formation of a softer, more flocculent curd that can be more easily digested by the infant's enzymes. The dilution of milk has the advantage of creating a calcium concentration more near to human milk but reduces caloric concentration. Sucrose can be added to increase the calories.

During the first two weeks about 15 g sugar is added to the day's formula. Thereafter, 30 g is sufficient. Sugar is discontinued at the time the baby is taking appreciable amounts of other foods.

At two months the infants take about 120 ml of formula. This is increased by 30 ml every month until the infant is taking a maximum of 240 ml at approximately 6 months of age. Formula fed babies should not, as a rule be fed at less than 3 hour intervals since the cow's milk remains for a longer time in the stomach.

Different Strategies

Milk, bottle and other equipment should be sterilised before use. The feeding is usually warmed to body temperature or can be fed cold. As with breast feeding the baby should be held in a semi-reclining position. Tne hole in the nipple should not be large or too small. The nipple should be filled with fluid and not air. The baby should not be expected to finish the entire amount of formula in the bottle at each feeding. Proprietary formulas are available in dry form. Specified quantity of water is added to make up the volume.

Growth failure due to repeated infections or over diluting the formula, infantile obesity, iron deficiency anaemia, hypernatremia, neonatal hypocalcaemia, amino acidaemias in premature infants and acrodermatitis and enteropathica have all been reported. There is a higher prevalence of allergic disorders, infective morbidity, emotional instability and sudden death syndrome in bottle fed than in breast-fed infants.

Table below gives undesirable effect of cow's milk on human infant.

Preterm Baby : The preterm babies are those who are born before 37 weeks of gestation. Low birth weight babies are born with a birth weight of less than 2500 g. The incidence of low birth weight babies in India is 30 per cent.

The possible reasons for low birth weight of babies are low maternal body mass index, low age at marriage, low maternal nutritional status with respect to iron and folic acid and shorter duration of full term gestation.

The feeding is one of the major challenges in the care of the low birth weight babies. Goal of feeding the preterm is to achieve a growth rate that approaches the normal growth rate of foetus in utero.

Undesirable effect of Cow's Milk on Human Infant

Composition	*Undesirable effect*
* Low level of Lactose	* Reduced calcium absorption.
* High protein	* In small infants as the gut is not mature enough, there is chance for unsplit protein to escape into the circulation and cause sensitisation.
* Cow's milk protein intolerance	* Lactoglobulin or alpha casein may cause diarrhoea, respiratory allergy and eczema.
* Low osmolarity	* There is an increased additional load on immature kidney. Due to increased demand for water to excrete. This solute load, there is a chance for dehydration and constipation.

Contd...

Composition	Undesirable effect
* High levels of tyrosine	* Lead to azotemia and acidosis and aromatic amino acids that are not utilised
* SDA high	* Increased energy waste.
* High fat	* Infantile obesity.
* Low amount of iron and	* Iron deficiency anaemia, poor availability.
Enteric loss of blood	
Low Vitamin C	
* High Phosphate	* Decreased iron and calcium absorption.

The preterm is at a disadvantage in many aspects of nutrition. The problem facing the preterm are, poor sucking and swallowing reflexes, relatively high caloric requirement with small stomach capacity, poor gag reflex and incompetent cardio oesophageal sphincter leading to aspiration, decreased absorption of essential nutrients.

Nutritional Requirements Calories : The caloric need of non-growing preterm babies during the first week of life are 60 kcal/kg/day. After first one or two weeks of life most preterm babies require 120-150 kcal/kg/day to maintain satisfactory growth. High calories may be necessary in babies who are not gaining weight, post-operative patients and extreme pre-terms.

Fluid : Fluid needs of the preterm babies are relatively high during the first week of life. The intake of fluids varies from 90-100 ml/kg/day for 7-10 days. Additional fluids may be required when the baby is under the phototherapy or a radiant warmer.

Carbohydrate : Preterm babies can tolerate 50 per cent of the calories in the form of carbohydrates. Very low birth weight babies may have difficulty in tolerating the lactose the first few days. Glucose polymers are well tolerated.

Protein : Preterm babies require 3-4 g of protein per kilogram of body weight for rapid growth. Excess of protein may lead to metabolic problems of acidosis and hyperammonemia. Human milk contains mainly whey protein which are better utilised. Certain amino acids essential for the preterm such as cystine, taurine, alanine and arginine are present in breast milk.

Fat : Fat malabsorption and steatorrhoea can occur in preterms due to reduced amounts of pancreatic lipase, carboxylic ester hydrolase, bile acids and lingual lipase.

About 40-50 per cent of calories in diet of the preterm should be available from fats. Very low birth weight babies poorly digest and absorb saturated triglycerides. Vegetable oils containing unsaturated long chain fatty acids are better absorbed . Better still are medium chain triglycerids because their digestion and absorption are not dependent on bile salts level.

Minerals and Vitamins : Calcium and phosphorus supplements may be needed to prevent rickets or osteopenia in preterms. Iron deficiency can occur by 6-12 weeks and hence 2.5 mg/kg/day of iron starting from 6-8 weeks of age may be given. Zinc supplementation has been shown to increase weight gain. Zinc is found to be low in banked milk.

All low birth weight babies should receive vitamin supplementation in addition to the amount present in human milk. This is because :

(a) Premature infants are born with low body stores of vitamin,

(b) Their growth rates are rapid,

(c) Their gastrointestinal absorption is reduced, and

(d) Their daily intake of milk feedings is initially low. Table below shows the nutritional supplements required for preterm babies.

Feeding the Preterm Baby : The preterm babies are best fed with unprocessed human milk obtained from their mothers. It has been shown that milk of mothers delivering prematurely has higher caloric, fat, protein and sodium content which is suitable for the nutritional needs of low birth weight babies. Antimicrobial property of breast milk is of great importance to the preterm baby. If the baby does not gain weight satisfactorily with breast milk alone, dietary supplements like vegetable oils (corn oil, groundnut oil) may be used which increase the caloric value without increasing its volume.

When human milk feeding is not possible one must resort to animal milk or formula feeds. Formula milk for preterm are now being introduced in India.

Nutritional Supplements of Preterm Babies

Nutrient	*Amount*	*Frequency*
Vitamin AI.U	1000	Orally after two weeks
Vitamin C mg	35	Orally after two weeks
Vitamin DI.U	400	Orally after two weeks
Folic acid mcg	50	Orally after two weeks
Vitamin K mg	0.5 -1	At birth and biweekly if infant is receiving TPN or antibiotics
Vitamin EI.U	15	If the infant weight is less than 1500 g this should be given for 36 weeks.
Zinc mg/kg	800-1200	If breast milk is not given this supplementation is needed.
Iodine mg./kcal	4.5	-do-
Copper mcg./kg/day	100-200	-do-
Sodium mcg./kg	4.8	-do-

The decision whether a baby is to be breast fed or through a gavage is guided by maturity, birth weight and general condition of the baby. The infant can be started with expressed mother's milk. Bolus, intermittent, naso-gastric tube feeds every 2 hours in small babies and every 3 hours in larger babies can be done. Initial volume used will be as low as 1-2 ml for feeding infants of 1000 g or less or as much as 4-5 ml per feed for an infant of 1500 g.

If oral feeds are tolerated, then increase the volume of feeding by 1 ml/day in smaller infants or by as much as 3-5 ml in the larger infants. Feeding must be reduced, withheld or even omitted entirely when there is gastric retention or abdominal distension. Ultimately the volume of intake should be 150-170 ml/kg/day and caloric value 110-120 ml/kg/day. If the rate of weight gain is low the caloric intake is increased by adding vegetable oil (coconut oil or peanut oil, 0.5 ml every other feed). Most infants begin to gain more rapidly as their postnatal weight approaches 1400-1500 g and their caloric intake increases.

The preterm infant's poor nutritional reserves, high requirements for normal growth and development, and gastrointestinal immaturity pose a particularly challenging nutritional problem. Nutritional programme should be given a high priority in the overall care of preterm infants.

Difficulties Ahead

Underfeeding: Underfeeding is suggested by restlessness and crying and by failure to gain weight adequately, despite complete emptying of the breast or bottle. Underfeeding may also result from the infant's failure to take a sufficient quantity of food even when offered. Constipation, failure to sleep, irritability and excess crying can result due to underfeeding.

Diarrhoea : Diarrhoea in a breast fed infant is unusual. Mild diarrhoeal disturbances due to over feeding respond quickly to temporary decrease or cessation of feeding. Withholding all solid food as well as one or several milk feedings and substituting boiled water or a balanced electrolyte solution are usually all that is required.

Constipation : Constipation in the artificially fed infant may be caused by an insufficient amount of food or fluid. In other cases, it may result from diets too high in fat or protein or deficient in bulk. Simply increasing the amount of fluid or sugar in the formula may be corrective in the first few months of life. After this age, better results are obtained by adding or increasing the amounts of cereal, vegetables and fruits.

Colic: The term colic describes a frequent symptom complex of paroxysmal abdominal pain, presumably of intestinal origin and of severe crying. It occurs usually in infants younger than 3 months.

Prevention of attacks should be sought by improving feeding techniques, including burping, providing a stable emotional environment, identifying possibly allergemic foods in the infant's or nursing mother's diet and avoiding underfeeding or overfeeding.

Weaning : The term "weaning" comes from the word "wemian" which means to accustom. Weaning begins from the moment supplementary food is started and continues till the child is taken off the breast completely. Solid food added to an infant's diet is called beikost. There is an increase in activities of the enzymes at the time of weaning.

Need for Weaning : Infants in our country thrive on breast milk alone up to six months of life and their growth rate during this period is satisfactory. Breast milk alone is not able to provide sufficient amounts of all the nutrients needed to maintain growth after the first six months. Increasing needs of calories and protein of growing children cannot be met by the diminishing output of mother's milk. Milk is also a poor source of vitamin C and supplementation with fruit juice is essential. Iron stores in liver of the infant would last only upto 4-6 months. Hence iron-rich foods should be given at least from six months onwards.

Milk is also deficient in vitamin D. If the baby is to maintain the expected rate of growth and remain healthy and well nourished, supplementary feeding has to be resorted to round about the 6th month of life.

Results of some of the investigations conducted at National Institute of Nutrition, Hyderabad, suggest that early introduction of supplements before six months of age is not associated with any beneficial effect on infant growth. It is possible that introduction of supplements results in reduction in suckling stimulus and therefore reduction in milk output resulting in shorter duration of lactation and shorter duration of lactational amenorrhoea and inter-pregnancy interval.

Though Indian babies are given supplementary foods, either they are introduced very late or given adult form of diet. The age of introduction of supplementation is 3-5 months in the urban elite and middle income group. The supplementation is delayed in urban poor by 7-9 months and rural poor by 9-11 months.

Introduction of weaning food too late can lead to undernutrition and increased diarrhoeal morbidity.

Bulky adult diet, when given to infants, usually does not meet the nutritional requirement, particularly calories. Nutrient density of weaning foods of western diet is 1.0 kcal/g of food whereas in Asia, the nutrient density is 0.25 kcal to 0.4 kcal/g. Hence calorie dense foods like malted food should be given to infants. Weaning food should provide at least 10% of the energy as protein.

Types of Supplementary Foods

Liquid Supplements

Milk : At about the sixth month of life the frequency of breast feeding is reduced to 3 or 4 times per day and animal milk is substituted. Since the proportion of nutrients in animal milk differs from that of human milk, the cow's milk is diluted with boiled and cooled water in the proportion of 2:1 for the first feeds. The amount of water is gradually reduced so that in the course of a few weeks the baby receives undiluted animal milk. Two feeds, with 225 ml of milk per feed is an ideal replacement. Sugar can be added for taste and to increase calories.

Juice of Fresh Fruits : Oranges, tomatoes, sweet lime, grapes serve to supplement the protective nutrients not present in sufficient amounts in breast milk as well as in animal milk. It is advantageous to start feeding small quantities of fresh fruit juice even in the 3rd or 4th month of life.

In the early stages, the fruit juice is diluted with an equal amount of boiled water and only a couple of teaspoonfuls are fed. The amount of fruit juice fed is gradually increased and at the same time the dilution with water is cut down. In a week's time the baby receives 85 ml orange juice or about 170 ml fresh tomato juice. Since tomato juice does not contain the same proportion of nutrients as orange juice, double the quantity is required.

Soup from Green Leafy Vegetables : In case fresh fruits are not available, green leafy vegetables may be used as an alternative. Strained soup can be given in the beginning with unstrained soup later on.

Fish Liver Oil : Fish liver oils are good source of vitamin A and D. Infants should be given a few drops to 1/2 tsp per day mixed in small quantity of milk.

Solid Supplements Mashed well before Feeding : Mashed food is started around the 7th or 8th month of life. Around this time, the infant is already receiving animal milk, fruit juice or vegetable soup and fish liver oil.

Cereal and Starchy Gruels : To meet the increasing demands of calories and protein, well cooked mashed cereals mixed with milk and sugar can be given. Calorie dense cereals can be prepared using malted wheat or ragi.

Preparation of Malted Cereal : Soak the cereal overnight. Remove the water and tie in a moist cloth and keep in warm place. After 48 hours when sprouts come out, dry in sun or roast it. Remove the sprouts as there may be toxic substances in the sprouts. Make into flour.

During the process of malting, starch is converted to maltose due to increased production of enzyme amylase. This is also called Amylase Rich Food. Due to the conversion of starch into amylose, thinner gruels are made. With this either the infant can consume more gruel or more flour can be added to make thick gruel. This way calorie consumption can be increased.

Other cereals like, rice, rice flour, rice flakes, corn flakes, can also be given in the form of porridge.

Vegetables : Cooked, mashed vegetables like potato, green leafy vegetables and carrots can be introduced to get vitamins and minerals and colours in the diet.

Fruits : All fruits, with the exception of banana which is mashed, must be stewed and sieved for one year old baby. Thereafter, it is given simply stewed, with the addition of a little sugar and lime juice for flavour.

Non-vegetarian Foods : A small amount of hard boiled yolk of egg is given to start with and if the infant tolerates, the amount may be gradually increased to a complete yolk of an egg. Yolk is a good source of vitamin A, iron and protein. Soft custard is also a suitable way in which to introduce egg yolk. Egg white, because of the frequency of allergic manifestations, is not given until the infant is 8 to 10 months old and then it is given very cautiously. The whole egg may be poached or soft boiled and fed by the time the baby reaches the age of one year.

Finally, minced and cooked meat or boiled fish may be fed after suitably flavouring with salt, 3 to 4 times a week.

Pulses : Well cooked pulses along with cereals in the form of Khichdi/ pongal can be given or can be made into porridge. Pulse and meat preparations can be given at alternate days.

Solid Supplements Unwashed : When the baby starts cutting his teeth, it is time to start chopped and lumpy foods. Cooked cereals, pulses and vegetables can be given to the child. Solids like idli, idiappam, bread, Chapati, rice and dal can be given after the child gets used to semi-solids.

Vegetables may be chopped into small pieces, and boiled. Cooked potato can be given. After a year, leafy vegetables can be given well boiled and soft. A slice of raw carrot or fruit segments with all skin and seeds removed is a good exercise for the gums. As the child grows, it is better to give fruit segments instead of juice. Fruit provides bulk in the diet and is good for bowel movement.

Points to be Considered

- Introduce only one food at a time.
- Allow the infant to become familiar with the food before trying to give another.
- Give very small amounts of any new food at the beginning, for example, one tea spoon full or less.
- Use a very thin consistency when starting solid foods. Gradually the consistency is made more solid as the infant learns to propel the food back with the help of tongue.

- If, after several trials, the baby has an acute dislike for a particular food, omit that item for a week or two and then try again. If the dislike persists it is better to forget about the food for a while and substitute another.
- Food should be only slightly seasoned.
- At first strained fruits, vegetables and cereals are given.
- When the baby is able to chew, gradually substitute finely chopped fruits and vegetables usually at 8 to 9 months.
- Infants may object to taking some foods by themselves but will take them willingly if one is mixed with another, e.g., egg may be mixed with formula, cereal or vegetable. Vegetables may sometimes be made into soup with little milk until the baby becomes accustomed to the new flavour.
- Variety in choice of foods is important.
- The mother or anyone feeding the infant must be careful to avoid showing in any way a dislike for a food which is being given.
- A baby's appetite varies a lot from meal to meal and day to day. During hot weather or when the child is teething or suffering from cold the child's appetite may be less.
- Give freshly prepared food.
- To make the food calorie dense add oil, butter or ghee to the infant's
- Fruit juice should be fed only by cup not by bottle.

Feeding an infant with supplementary foods demands greater skill and ingenuity on the part of the mother than the mere selection of suitable foods and cooking them in suitable ways. To guide the child to learn to eat and enjoy foods, the mother must be patient, resourceful and not too serious.

By one year, the infant can be given family diet, modified, in small quantities but at frequent intervals in addition to milk. The best indication of adequacy of the diet is the growth pattern of the child.

Low Cost Supplementary Food : Indian mothers wean their infants into the traditional adult diet because of their ignorance of low cost weaning foods and also because of incapacity to buy expensive commercial foods.

Table below gives a list of some of the low cost nutritious supplementary foods which can be given by the poor mothers of the slum and rural areas to their infants.

Instant ready to use infant foods are standardised at Coimbatore (cereal 30 g, pulse 20 g, roasted ground nuts 10 g and jaggery 15 g). NIN Hyderabad (bajra/ragi 60 g, green gram dal 15 g, skim milk powder 10 g, til 5 g, sugar or salt to taste) and at Gandhigram (ground nut cake biscuits, ragi biscuits).

Problems in Weaning

Obesity : Too early and too much quantity of feeding or too concentrated food can lead to over weight of the infant.

Underweight : Too less quantity of food and less concentrated foods can lead to underweight. Bulky adult food, when consumed by an infant gives satiety without meeting calorie requirement. This results in underweight of the child. Frequent illness and repeated diarrhoeas can also result in underweight of the child.

Allergy : The foods most frequently implicated in infant allergies are wheat, milk, egg and citrus juices. Rice is probably the most hypoallergenic of the commonly eaten cereals. The consumption of wheat is best delayed until after the 6th month. Egg white, which is a potent sensitiser is usually deferred until the 10th month. Egg yolk is less allergenic and heat denaturation renders egg yolks non-reactive. The pure orange juice does not arouse allergic reactions in infants or children. Improperly prepared orange juice may contain excessive amounts of peel oil or of seed proteins which have leached into the juice from broken seeds and may therefore cause reactions in susceptible children.

Allergy to milk is the most serious of the commonly encountered food allergies since milk supplies the basic nutritional requirements in early infancy. In most cases the allergic reaction is due to the presence of lacto-globulins and to some extent lactoalbumin. The infant can be fed evaporated milk in which these proteins are denatured.

In most cases, food protein allergy is transitory. Tolerance is achieved in 50 per cent by the end of first year and 80 per cent after three years. Artificial flavours and colours have been associated with respiratory allergic disorder.

Low Cost Supplementary Foods Developed in India

Name of the product	*Composition*
• Indian multipurpose food (C.F.T.R.I)	Low fat groundnut flour and bengal gram flour (75 : 25) fortified with vitamins A and D, B_1, B_2 and calcium carbonate. Contains 42 per cent protein.
• Malt food (C.F.T.R.I)	Cereal malt, low fat groundnut flour, roasted bengal gram flour (40 : 40 : 20) fortified with vitamins and calcium salts. Contains 28 per cent protein.
• Balahar (C.F.T.R.I)	Whole wheat flour, groundnut flour and roasted bengal gram flour (70 :20 :10) fortified with calcium salts and vitamins. Contains 20 per cent protein.
• Supplementary food (N.I.N)	Roasted wheat flour, green gram flour, groundnut and sugar or jaggery. (30 :20 : 8 : 20). Contains 12.5 per cent proteins.
• Supplementary food (A.H.S.C.W.) Kuzhandai Amudhu	Roasted maize flour, green gram flour, roasted groundnut and jaggery (30 :20:10:20). Contains 14.4 per cent proteins.
• Win food (Gandhigram Rural Institute)	Pearl millet, green gram dal, groundnut flour, and jaggery (50:15:25:25). Contains 20 per cent proteins.

Contd...

Name of the product	*Composition*
• Amutham	Rice flour, ragi flour, bengal gram flour, sesame flour, groundnut flour and jaggery (15:15:15:10:10:25). Contains 14 per cent proteins.
• Poshak	Cereal (wheat, maize, rice or jowar) pulse (chana dal or green gram dal) and oil seed (groundnut) and jaggery (4:2:1:2).
• Poshak (least cost weaning mix)	Same ingredients as poshak but in the proportion of 60 :17 :14: 9
• Kerala Indigenous Food (KIF)	Tapioca, Bulgar wheat and groundnut (25 : 50 :25)

Refusal to Take New Food : If the child refuses to take new food, form of the food can be modified or should be mixed with the food he likes and should be tried again after a week or so. Frequently a child may spit out the first spoon of food but usually this means that he does not know how to swallow the non-liquid food.

Choking : Choking and aspiration can be caused by peanuts, seeds, small hard sweets, crisps and raisins. Hard and big pieces of fruit like apple or vegetable popcorn should be avoided for children under 3 years of age since they can cause choking which can lead to death.

Some Suggested Recipes during Infancy

Recipe	*Reason*
Fruit juice (4 months)	Provides vitamin C which is lacking in milk. Tomato and orange juice also supply some amount of beta carotene.
Greens soup (6 months)	Child gets used to new taste, provides iron, calcium, beta carotene, riboflavin and vitamin C.

Contd...

Recipe	*Reason*
Stewed apple (8 months)	Gives calories and should not be given in raw pieces since it may choke the child.
Soft custard with egg yolk (8 months)	Provides vitamin A, iron, protein and B vitamins. Egg white should be introduced later as it may cause allergy.
Khichdi (pongal), idli, Chapati + milk, (10-12 months)	Easily digestible and gives calories and good quality protein.
Malted cereals and gruels made out of rice, rice flour, rice flakes, corn flakes and milk.	Meets increased demands of calories and protein.

7

Diet for Children

Early Phase

The years between 1 and 6, growth is generally slower than in the first year of life but continues gradually. Activity also increases markedly during the second year of life as the child becomes increasingly mobile. Development of a full dentition by about the age of 2 years also increases the range of foods that can safely be eaten. There is an increased need for all nutrients, but the pattern of increase varies for different nutrients in relation to their role in growth of specific tissues.

Food Requirements

Energy : Energy is required for growth and activity. Insufficient food will not only result in undernutrition in terms of inadequate weight gain but will also hinder growth. The rate of growth fluctuates from one age to another. Upto 10 years of age there is no difference in sex for RDA. Due to improper weaning practices, the child may not meet calorie and protein requirement and pave the way for PEM. Insufficient calorie intake can lead to protein deficiency.

Proteins : The increase in the muscle mass that must accompany bone growth requires positive nitrogen balance that is met by protein intake of 1.5 to 2 g/kg body weight. The increase in total body size necessitates a larger vascular system to transport nutrients to the tissues and waste all products away from the tissues. Thus there is an increase in demand for nutrients needed in blood formation like protein, iron, folacin and pyridoxine. Bone growth also creates a need for protein.

The RDA of pre-school children (1-6 years) is given in Table below.

Recommended Dietary Allowances for Pre-school Children

Nutrient	*Years* 1-3	4-6
Weight kg.	12.2	19.0
Energy k cal	1240	1690
Protein g	22	30
Fat g	25	25
Calcium mg	400	400
Iron mg	12	18
Vitamin A mcg	400	400
Beta carotene mcg	1600	1600
Thiamine mg	0.6	0.9
Riboflavin mg	0.7	1.0
Nicotinic acid mg	8	11
Pyridoxine mg	0.9	0.9
Ascorbic acid mg	40	40
Folic acid mcg	30	40
Vitamin B_{12} mcg	0.2 to 1	0.2 to 1

Fat : Fat energy including invisible fat for children should be 25 per cent of total energy and essential fatty acid energy is 5-6 per cent.

Minerals : Calcium requirements of children is calculated on the basis of the amount of calcium accretion in the body. This deposition is not uniform throughout growing period, but would be relatively greater during early childhood and during adolescence than during the other periods of growth. Since, all dietary calcium is not absorbed 400 mg/day is prescribed though the actual requirement may be less. Deficiency of calcium can affect the bones of growing children. Milk is the best source of calcium. Hence the diet of pre-school child should include 1-2 glasses of milk per day.

During growth for an increase in each kilogram in body weight 30 mg of iron is required and since the increase in body weight during childhood is 2 kg/year on an average, the daily requirement of iron for growth will be 0.2 mg. The physiological requirement can vary markedly for 1-2 years from 0.2-0.5 mg per kg of body weight per day.

To meet this increased demand for iron, iron-rich foods like rice flakes, egg yolk and greens should be included in the diet. Dietary lack of iron accompanied by hookworm infestation can lead to anaemia.

Vitamins : The incidence of vitamin A deficiency signs are high and serum vitamin A levels are generally low among Indian children whose dietary intake is less than 100 mcg. According to the studies conducted by ICMR, children receiving food supplements which provided a total of 300 mcg of vitamin A per day over a period of 6 months, serum vitamin A levels were found to be around 30 mg/di and no clinical signs of vitamin A deficiency. Based on this data 400 mcg have been suggested including the safety allowances. Deficiency of vitamin A in children can cause bitot's spots, night blindness or in severe cases total blindness also. Milk, eggs, carrots and green leafy vegetables should be included in the diet.

A level of 200 I.U. of vitamin D is suggested purely tentatively as dietary allowances for Indian children.

The daily allowances of B-vitamin requirements are based on energy intake. The allowances per 1000 kcals are (same as an adult) 0.5 mg thiamine, 0.6 mg riboflavin and 6.6 mg niacin equivalents. Requirements for children for folic acid and B_{12} were computed from interpolation of values for infants and adults.

Elements at Work

Nearly two out of three pre-school children in India are malnourished.

Growth is influenced by nutrition. Frequent attacks of infectious diseases affect their growth and increase the requirements of various nutrients. Incidence of PEM and vitamin A deficiency are high among this age group.

Repeated illnesses—especially the common illnesses such as diarrhoea, measles, whooping cough and other respiratory infections—are the principal underlying causes of malnutrition. They take away appetite and so reduce food intake often for many days each month, they inhibit the absorption of the food that is eaten, they drain the body of nutrients through diarrhoea and vomiting, they burn up calories in fever. The result is frequent weight loss. The mechanisms by which infections worsen nutritional status are anorexia, cultural and therapeutic practices, malabsorption, catabolic losses, anabolic losses, fever, additional intestinal losses, reduced growth and weight loss.

Overall need for nutrients increases throughout the growth period but there will be periods when growth is slow and the need for certain nutrients will be reduced proportionately. Children reflect these changes in need, by fluctuations in appetite. This may cause anxiety to parents. Unless such period is prolonged or is accompanied by signs of undernutrition such as lethargy, fatigue and increased susceptibility to infection, should not cause concern.

Needs for Diets

Transition from infant diet to regular adult diet should be smooth and gradual. If solid foods have been gradually introduced before the age of one year, feeding the child should be no problem in the subsequent years. But some pre-schoolers are difficult eaters at times. Some children less than 5-6 years of age are finicky eaters. Moreover, many tend to use eating (or not eating) to exert control over parents.

Dietary Guidelines

- The diet should be adequate in quantity and quality of different nutrients. In addition to the amount of milk recommended, the pre-school child should have two small servings of protein-rich foods. When the child is about 18 months old, finger foods such as carrots can be given.

- Proper elimination is usually maintained by a daily diet of fruits, vegetables and whole grain products.
- The diet should include a variety of foods. The child who is taught to eat everything on his plate is much more likely to enjoy optimal health than is the one who picks and chooses. The child should have access to items from all food groups on a regular basis.
- Their food intake will improve if the food is interesting and attractive, e.g., Chapatis, puris can be made into shapes or can be served in attractive plates. Flavour or colour of the milk can be changed to encourage the child to drink more milk.
- Foods should be slightly seasoned so that they taste better and the child takes it well.
- Child should never be forced to eat more than he can take.
- The person feeding the child with the food should not show any dislike of that food in front of the child. This may lead to the rejection of food by the child.
- Children are sensitive to flavours, any change in flavour of daily food may lead to its rejection.
- Food preferences of the child should be taken into consideration.
- Regularity of meal times is essential.
- Different cooking methods and new attractive combinations encourage the child to eat more.
- The child should never be hurried while taking the food. The atmosphere should be pleasant, peaceful and lacking distraction.
- Foods like tea and coffee should be restricted as they overstimulate the system.

- The energy density should be 1.0 to 1.2 kcal/ml. This can be achieved by adding milk and oil to the diet. Malted foods can also be included in the diet to increase calorie density.
- Unripe bananas and apples should not be given as they are difficult to chew and may choke the child.

Even if there is enough food in the house to provide an adequate diet, growth can be faltered due to feeding a young child with bulky staple foods which fill the child's stomach and assuage its hunger without meeting its energy needs. Also feeding a child's small stomach infrequently (only twice instead of four times) can affect the growth of the child.

Special care is needed for feeding children below two years of age, since they cannot ask for food and have not yet learnt to eat by themselves.

Picky Eaters

* Accept a limited number of food choices.
* Are unwilling to take new foods.
* Avoid some food groups such as vegetables.
* Exhibit strong food preferences including presentation and preparations styles.

Picky eater phenomenon is independent of social status. Psychological and physiological problems need to be corrected.

Dental Problems of Pre-school Children : Tooth decay can be caused by caries. This can occur in children who are susceptible and whose integrity of tooth structure may be affected by the nutritional deficiency. Vitamin A is necessary for enamel and vitamin C is essential for dentine. Calcium, phosphorous and vitamin D are needed for the process of calcification. Flourine decreases susceptibility of caries.

Fermentable carbohydrate which adhers to the tooth surface is the major dietary factor influencing tooth decay. Stickier the carbohydrate and longer the sugar is in the mouth, the greater the cariogenic effect.

Suggested Recipes for Pre-school Children

Recipe	*Reasons*
Noodles	Give calories and the child enjoys the shape of it.
Tricolour sandwich (mint chutney, tomato sauce or jam)	Attractive, tempting to the child. Gives calories and vitamins.
Biscuits (different types and shapes)	Pre-school child identifies and enjoys in eating. Provides calories and proteins.
Milk shakes, fruit shakes, ice creams	Indirect form of consuming milk as the child may get bored to take plain milk.
Chikki	Crisp foods the child willingly consumes, calories protein and B-vitamins are the important nutrients the child gets from this.
Banana chips, wafers	Crisp foods the child likes.

Nutrition Related Problems : The primary cause of malnutrition is inadequate and faulty diet. Apart from poverty and other socio-economic factors, environmental factors also play an important role in aggravating the dietary deficiency diseases.

These precipitating factors are the widespread chronic infections among the poor living under conditions of poor environmental sanitation and personal hygiene. Thus a marginal intake of nutrients which by itself may not lead to clinical deficiency may do so when infectious diseases are superimposed.

The peak prevalence of kwashiorkor was frequently seen in the age group of 2-3 years and marasmus in 1-2 years. Over 80% of the under fives are estimated to be malnourished and around 1-2% suffer from severe malnutrition. Around 25% hospital beds are occupied by patients whose major problem is malnutrition. In more than 50% of deaths in children, malnutrition is the direct or indirect cause. PEM is a silent killer in many children.

The NNMB survey (1988-90) of rural children shows that only about 10 per cent are normal with weights above 90 per cent of the standard NCHS. A majority of them exhibit mild or moderate malnutrition while 7-8 per cent are severely malnourished.

Table below gives prevalence of malnutrition in preschool children and infants.

Prevalence of Malnutrition in Preschool Children and Infants

Aspects	*Prevalence%*
Low birth weight	30
Kwashiorkor/ Marasmus	1-2
Bitot's spot	3
Iron Deficiency anaemia	50
Underweight (weight for age)	53
Stunting (height for age)	65

About 1-2% of preschool children suffer from severe and florid forms of PEM like kwashiorkor and marasmus. Country wide surveys indicate that more than a half of the Indian preschool children (1-5 years) suffer from sub-clinical undernutrition as indicated by low weight for age. About 65% of them are stunted (low height for age) which indicates that under-nutrition is of long duration.

In the case of vitamin A deficiency, upto 3% of preschool children show Bitot's spots and night blindness and about 30-40 thousand children become blind every year. Vitamin A deficiency also increases the risk of disease and death. More than 50% of preschool children also suffer from anaemia.

Protein Energy Malnutrition : Protein Energy Malnutrition is defined as a range of pathological conditions arising from coincident lack of varying proportions of protein and calorie, occurring most frequently in infants and young children and often associated with infection (WHO 1973).

C. Gopalan, in 1971 did systematic diet survey and found that kwashiorkor and marasmic children consume similar diets and brought out the 'theory of adaptation'. Child reacts to the stress of PEM and secretes cortisol which mobilises protein from muscle and subcutaneous tissue to amino acid pool resulting in wasting with no oedema and no hepatomegaly. Raised cortisol level lowers growth hormone and so the child is stunted. Marasmus is said to be well adapted to the stress of deficit in protein and calories. Sometimes the child is not able to adapt to the stress of inadequate diet, infection and separation from mother due to subsequent pregnancy. In dysadaptation, the adrenal is unable to secrete cortisol and mobilisation of protein from muscle is not possible and liver cannot synthesise β lipo protein and fatty liver occurs. Dysadaptation occurs and the child will ultimately land up as kwashiorkor.

The prevalence rate of severe degree of PEM in our community is 3-5 per cent. For every 3 to 5 cases of severe PEM, we can detect 80-90 cases of mild to moderate PEM and about 10 per cent of well nourished children.

Systematic study of the habitual diets of these children indicated that the concentration of protein in their diets was adequate, but they were suffering from energy or food inadequacy since they were not eating enough of their habitual diet. The average energy deficit was found to be 300 kcal/day.

The following are the causes for underweight for age which may precipitate into PEM.

(a) Due to poverty, mother is not able to provide sufficient food to the child resulting in undernutrition. (b) The starchy gruels made from local staple food like rice, wheat, bajra, ragi, jowar or maize would result in "dietary bulk with a low caloric density". Hence the child may not be able to meet calorie requirement. Malted foods meet calorie requirement as they increase the caloric density, (c) Abrupt weaning, late weaning ignorance of importance of weaning can lead to undernutrition. (d) Malnutrition can result in less enzymes synthesis and less appetite leading to less consumption of food. (e) Chronic infections like primary complex may result in anorexia. (f) Infestation like ascariasis particularly giardiasis may lead to anorexia.

Symptoms of Different Types of PEM

Kwashiorkor : Oedema of the face and lower limbs, failure to thrive, anorexia, diarrhoea, apathy, dermatosis (hypo and hyper pigmentation) flaky paint appearance, sparse, soft and thin hair, angular stomatitis, cheilosis, and anaemia.

Marasmic Kwashiorkor : These children exhibit a mixture of some of the features of both marasmus and kwashiorkor.

Marasmus : Failure to thrive, irritability, fretfulness and apathy are common. Diarrhoea is frequent. Many are hungry but some may be anorexia. The child is shrunk and there is little or no subcutaneous fat. There is often dehydration. The temperature is subnormal. Watery diarrhoea and acid stools may be present. The muscles are weak and atrophic and this together with the lack of subcutaneous fat, makes the limbs appear as skin and bones.

Nutritional Dwarfing : Some children adapt to prolonged insufficiency of food-energy and protein—by a marked retardation of growth. Weight and height are both reduced resembling children a year or more younger.

The Underweight Child : These children are growing up smaller than their genetic potential and of greater importance as they are at risk of gastroenteritis, respiratory and other infections, which can precipitate frank malnutrition.

Clinical Features of Different Types of PEM : The clinical presentation depends on the type, severity and duration of dietary deficiencies. The five forms are summarised in Table.

Classification of PEM (FAO/WHO)

	Body weight as % of standard	*Oedema*	*Deficit in weight for height*
Kwashiorkor	80-60	+	+
Marasmic kwashiorkor	< 60	+	+ +
Marasmus	< 60	0	+ +
Nutritional dwarfing	< 60	0	minimal
Underweight child	80-60	0	+

Nutritional Requirement in PEM : The diet should be rich in proteins of good quality and high in calories. The other nutritional requirements also must be met.

Energy : The child should be given 150 to 200 kcal/kg/body weight/day for the existing weight. For children less than 2 years 200 kcal/kg body weight should be given and for older children 150 to 175 kcal/kg body weight. It is very important that there should be enough calories in the diet, otherwise proteins will be utilised for energy purposes and not for building the tissues. Malted cereals can also be given to increase calorie density. Fifty per cent of total calories can be from carbohydrate.

Protein : Five grams of protein/kg body weight/day should be given for the existing weight (e.g., Weight of the child-5 kg. Requirement of protein is 25 g). The calories derived from protein should be 10 per cent of the total calculated calories per day if the main source is animal protein. If the main and the only source is from cereal and pulse then the percentage of calories derived from protein can be 13 to 14 per cent of the total calories because of the net protein utilisation of cereal and pulses is around 60 per cent whereas milk or egg is around 90 per cent. Though vegetable protein is as good as milk protein in reversing the acute manifestations of kwashiorkor, they are inferior in their ability to promote regeneration of serum albumin. This can be overcome by giving 3 parts of vegetable protein to one part of animal protein like skim milk.

Fats : Forty per cent of total calories can be from fat which can be tolerated by children. Saturated fats such as butter, milk and coconut oil are preferred because unsaturated fatty acids worsen diarrhoea.

Treatment : Treatment strategy can be divided into three stages:

- Resolving life-threatening conditions.
- Restoring nutritional status without disrupting homeostasis.
- Ensuring nutritional rehabilitation.

Criteria for Improvement

- Disappearance of mental apathy in 4 to 5 days.
- Disappearance of oedema in 7 to 10 days.
- Weight gain in 3 to 4 weeks.
- Rise in serum albumin level in about 2 weeks time.

There are three stages of treatment—hospital treatment, dietary management and rehabilitation.

Proper Healthcare

Hypothermia : Hypothermia, hypoglycaemia and gram negative sepsis often go together.

The child should be kept warm and practised " bedding in" with the mother.

Hypoglycaemia : In sick children, 10% dextrose 4 ml/kg should be followed by 10% dextrose as maintenance fluid with one ml Kcl for each 100 ml of IV fluid. Oral feeding should be initiated as early as possible.

Septicaemia/Infections : Broad spectrum antibiotics, crystalline penicillin or ampicillin with an aminoglycoside should be given. Staphylococcal infections should also be treated.

Dehydration and Electrolyte Imbalance : In children with diarrhoea, if there is no dehydration, half to one glass of ORS or home available fluid (HAF) to prevent dehydration after each stool should be given. In mild to moderate dehydration, 70 ml/kg ORS in 4 hours, sip by sip or as intra gastric drip should be given. In severe dehydration 100 ml/kg N saline or Ringer Lactate (RL) in 3 to 6 hours should be given. In oedematous children 70 ml/kg should be given as a slow ration. Half the calculated fluid can be given as NS/RL and the rest as 10% glucose. This will tackle hypoglycaemia and will reduce sodium intake. They usually have hypokalaemia and so add Kcl 1 to 2 ml to each 100 ml of IVF. Potassium supplement, 2-4 mEq/kg/day may be continued for 12 weeks in Kwashiorkor 15% IV Kcl will give 2mEq/ml and 1.5 ml oral Kcl will give 2 mEq. Fruit juice can be encouraged to supplement potassium. Sodium should be restricted to 2-3 mEq/day. If there is evidence of acidosis, sodium bicarbonate 2ml/kg IV diluted with equal quantity of distilled water should be given.

Heart Failure : In case of heart failure, fluid intake should be two third of the maintenance and frusemide 1-2 mg/kg should be given. If diuretic therapy is needed for more than a day in addition to potassium supplementation aldactone 2-3 mg/kg/day. Oedema of kwashiorkor is not treated by diuretics.

Anaemia : Severe anaemia should be corrected by small packed cell transfusion, 5-10 ml/kg slowly along with fursemide. In mild to moderate anaemia, start 6 mg/kg of elemental iron is given after the patient has been stabilised and preferably after deworming.

Vitamin and Mineral Deficiencies : In vitamin A deficiency and in all florid cases of PEM 2 lakh IU of vitamin A is given. For infants, the dose is 1 lakh IU. The dose may be repeated after one day or one month and also initiate them into the vitamin A prophylaxis programme. Vitamin K 2-5 mg IM/IV per day may be given for 2-3 days in florid PEM and in those with persistent diarrhoea. All B complex, vitamin C, K, D, zinc and calcium need to be supplemented. Magnesium is given if there is seizure tetany or apathy. Upto 0.8 m Eq/ kg/ day in 2 divided doses is given for 1-3 days.

Restoring Nutritional Status : This phase is for restoration of weight for height. This is the second and often the first step in those with mild to moderate PEM.

ORS	High Energy Milk	Milk 100 ml	= 600 kal
		Sugar 1 tsp	= 20 kal
		Oil ½ tsp	= 20 kcal
		Total 100 ml	= 100 kcal
Milk	Cereal milk	Milk 100 ml	= 60 kcal
		Sugar 1 tsp	= 20 kcal
		Cereal flour 1 ½ tsp	= 20
		Total 100ml	= 100 kcal
Family	Cereal pulse	Milk 100 ml	= 60 kcal
pot	milk	Sat Mix 2 tsp	
feeding		(Cereal+pulse+sugar)	= 40
		Total 100 ml	= 100 kcal

Nutritional Therapy in PEM

ORS followed by dilute milk, whole milk, high energy milk and high energy cereal milk can be given. To make high energy milk add 1 tsp sugar and ½ tsp coconut oil, to 100 ml milk in order to give 100 kcal/100 ml. Cereal flour or cereal pulse combination also may be added to 100 ml of high energy milk to make a thickened feed. A precooked ready to mix cereal pulse combination can be easily prepared at home by roasting and powdering rice, wheat, blackgram and adding powdered sugar in the ratio 1:1:1:2. This mix can be given as a semisolid mixed with hot water hot milk.

This mix is a research and development product of nutrition clinic department of paediatrics, SAT hospital, Medical college, Trivandrum and is named SAT mix. 100 g of this mix supplies 380 kcals and 8 g protein. Oil supplementation can be upto 10-15% of the calculated calories. Coconut oil is preferred as it is easily available, acceptable and has the advantage of the medium chain triglyceride. MCT is absorbed even during fat malabsorption.

Multivitamins and micronutrient should be started early. Once stable deworming should be done. Iron therapy is not initiated till carrier proteus are synthesised. Otherwise E. Coli will thrive on the unbound iron in the gut.

As a next step traditional food items such as rice, idli, uppama, tubers, legumers, payasam, egg, fish, green leafy vegetables, seasonal fruits etc. should be introduced gradually ensure family pot feeding as early as possible ground nuts can be given to be older children.

A weight gain of 0.5 g/week in children and 70 g/kg week in infant is the target but it us difficult to achieve if intercurrent infections occur frequently Restoration of weight for height may take about 8-12 weeks. Oedema clears and social smile returous in 1-2 weeks. Returns of social smile in severe PEM is an early sign of recovery.

8

Diet for Young Ones

During Childhood

The school-age period has been called the latent time of growth. The rate of growth slows and body changes occur gradually. Girls usually out distance boys by the latter part of this period.

The slowed rate of growth during this period results in a gradual decline in the food requirement per unit of body weight.

Food Requirements

The RDA of school children aged 6-12 years is given in Table below :

Recommended Dietary Allowances of School Children

Nutrient	*Years*		
	7-9	*10-12 boys*	*girls*
Weight kg	26.9	35.4	31.5
Energy kcal	1950	2190	1970
Protein g	41	54	57
Fat g	25	22	22

Contd...

Nutrient	*7-9*	*Years 10-12 boys*	*girls*
Calcium mg	400	600	600
Iron mg	26	34	19
Vitamin A mcg	600	600	600
β Carotene mcg	2400	2400	2400
Thiamine mg	1.0	1.1	1.0
Riboflavin mg	1.2	1.3	1.2
Nicotinic acid mg	13	15	13
Pyridoxine mg	1.6	1.6	1.6
Ascorbic acid mg	40	40	40
Folic acid mcg	60	70	70
Vitamin B_{12} mcg	0.2-1	0.2-1	0.2-1

Nutritional requirements of boys and girls are more or less the same till the first 9 years. After that, there is a variation in some nutrients.

Calories and Protein : Body requirements of calories are increased steadily for this age group. Requirements remain almost same for girls from 7-12 years. Requirements for boys are increased from 7-9 to 10-12 years as there is gradual increase in need because reserves are being laid down for the demands of the approaching adolescent period. The increased requirements of protein would meet demands of growth. Girls require more protein between 10-12 than boys for approaching menarche.

Minerals : Ten- to twelve-year old children require more calcium than adults to meet skeletal growth demands.

As the blood volume is increased iron requirements are also increased for boys. In childhood, from the second birthday to the twelfth in the male and the tenth in the female, the mean increase in body weight is 2.5-2.7 kg/year, equivalent to an iron requirement of 0.3 mg/day. The daily requirement is further increased by a rise in the haemoglobin concentration by about 1 g per decilitre. The amount of iron required to replace losses gradually increases from 0.2 mg/day during infancy to 0.5 mg/day in the twelfth year.

The requirement is lower in 10-12 year girls because of higher absorption - 5 per cent against 3 per cent in 7-9 year olds.

Vitamins : Vitamin A requirements of the children have been computed from the requirement figures for infants (50 *ug/kg)* and adults 9.3 ug/kg taking into account growth rates at different ages. The RDA of vitamin A and C are same as adult RDA. B-vitamin requirements are in proportion to calorie requirements.

Requirements of Food : There is an increasing interest and participation in other activities which compete with meal times. The important relationship of sound nutrition and learning has long been established. Breakfast is particularly important for a school child. It breaks the fast of the sleep hours and prepares a child for problem solving and memory spans in the learning period at school. Children who skip breakfast do not make up for nutrient and energy deficits later in the day and tend to perform more poorly on tests of cognition than those who eat breakfast. The school lunch programme provides a nourishing noon meal for many children who would not otherwise have one.

While eating with other children at school, the child observes many food attitudes and tastes new foods that he may not normally accept. The school-age child has increasing exposure to influence on food habits. Television also influences children in food selection. There are positive learning opportunities in the classroom, particularly when parents provide support at home and nutrition is integrated in academic activities. Many children tend to use eating or not eating to exert control over parents or caretakers.

The diet should contain from all Basic Five Food Groups. If the child does not have access to items from all food groups on a regular basis, self- selection of a balanced diet either within a day or over several days is impossible.

Making Healthful Choices : As children grow up, they became more independent about choosing their food. Children can be made to make healthful choices by :

- being a role model
- making them plant vegetables or fruit trees (children take pride in eating foods they have grown)
- taking them to farmer's market.
- allowing them to plan the dinner menu with the help of food guide pyramid.
- encouraging them to prepare simple recipes (They are more likely to fiat foods they have prepared).

Dietary Guidelines

- Nutritional requirement should meet their increasing activity and growth and special requirements because of sickness or injury.
- Children are generally restless and do not like to spend too much time at the table for eating. Besides, they feel rushed in the morning because they must reach their classes on time. So menus have to provide dishes that are quick to eat and yet satisfying nutritionally.
- Children also tend to be bored with foods easily. So menus need to provide variety in colour, texture, taste and flavour.
- The climatic and weather conditions are important consideration too. In hot weather extra liquids and salts are to be given because children do not generally like to drink plain water.
- Children have varying appetites and often prefer snacky meals at frequent intervals to a few large ones.
- New foods are likely to be accepted if it is given in a form which can be easily handled and they should be offered at regular intervals until the child learns to accept it.
- The young child should be encouraged to eat with the rest of the family as he is ready to take the family meals and also because the interactions between family members are a part of normal development.
- If the child does not like salads, they can be incorporated, in recipes like sandwiches.

Different Matters

Underweight : Many of our school children consume inadequate diet and so they are malnourished. Malnutrition can be due to poverty. Parents may not be able to provide nutritious food to their children. Sometimes ignorance on the part of parents to know the requirements of children quantitatively or qualitatively may lead to malnutrition of children.

When the child is in a hurry to go to school, he may miss breakfast or may not carry proper lunch to school or may become too tired after school activities and sleep off without taking night meal and thus skip the meals. Emotional disturbances at school due to poor academic performance or problems with siblings at home may reflect on the consumption of food.

Psychological factors contributing to depression or poor motivation to eat should be identified. Child's likes and dislikes need to be considered while feeding.

In order to overcome malnutrition in school children, sometimes government provides school lunch so that at least one-third of calorie and protein requirements are met.

Constipation : Children may not relish vegetables and fruits particularly green leafy vegetables. Parents should make an effort to motivate the child to eat by serving in different forms. Consumption of less quantity of food can lead to constipation. Early morning hurry to go to school and lack of sleep and activity can also lead to constipation.

Dental Caries : Consumption of sticky sweets can result in dental caries. Brushing the teeth before going to bed and after a meal should become a habit in children. Children should be encouraged to eat hard raw crisp foods.

Ready-made Food

Packed lunches have become a necessity for school going children as schools are either away or the lunch period is too short for the children to go home and have food. The packed lunch is a lunch that is packed in a tiffin box to be eaten by the child while away from home. It can be with one compartment or two or sometimes having more than 3 compartments.

Points to be Considered

- The packed lunch should meet one-third daily requirement of calories and protein of the child.
- Preferably, the packed lunch should consist of all five food groups, though the number of dishes may be less.
- Inclusion of one serving of green leafy vegetables would take care of one-third requirement of many vitamins and minerals.
- Some amount of good quality protein like milk or milk product like curd or paneer would improve vegetable protein. Or combination of vegetable proteins like cereals and pulses can be given for better utilisation. Addition of egg would also improve the quality of protein besides meeting many protective nutrient needs.
- To make the food appetizing, foods like whole fruit or butter milk in a bottle or chips in a polythene bag can be taken.
- Monotony should be avoided in packed lunches. There should be variety.
- It is sensible to have a different food in packed lunch than what one had for breakfast.
- The food should have the correct consistency. Too watery things may leak and too dry food may not be appetising to the child. Chapatis can be covered in cloth to retain moisture. Curd rice should be made with cold rice. Hot rice makes the water to separate from the curd.

Suggested Packed Lunches

Vegetable pulao, boiled egg, tomato raita and orange fruit.

Fenugreek leaves stuffed Chapati, thick dal and buttermilk.

Chapati stuffed with dal (thikada) with green leafy vegetables, sag.

Chapati, usal and carrot salad.

Cheese sandwiches or paneer sandwiches, guava.

Idli and kurma.

Dahi bada, tomato or cucumber slices and lemon pickle.

Khichdi, buttermilk, coriander chutney.

Sambar rice, amarnath porial, buttermilk.

Adai with drumstick leaves and coconut chutney.

Midday Meals

The school lunch programmes were started keeping in mind the social and economical advancement of the country. Urbanisation, industrialisation and an increase in the number of working mothers frequently brought about longer school days. This means, that children often did not receive proper meals at home and therefore needed to have a meal at school. Free compulsory primary education became more common and pressures were brought to bear on governmental authorities to provide school lunch.

Motives and Purposes

1. To provide food for undernourished children and to improve the nutritional status and monitor it.
2. To increase school enrolment and attendance of the children.
3. To reorient good eating habits.
4. To incorporate nutrition education into the curriculum.
5. To improve literacy and educational performance of the pupils.
6. To encourage the use of local commodities.
7. To encourage the community participation in the feeding programme.

Kitchen generally [illegible]

[illegible] and [illegible] pit.

[illegible] with drinking water and [illegible]

Midday Meals

The [illegible] conditions [illegible] to [illegible] and [illegible] of the [illegible] children [illegible] longer school days. [illegible] meals [illegible] compulsory primary education became more common and [illegible] brought [illegible] hunger.

Motives and Purposes

1. To provide food [illegible] education [illegible]

   (b) [illegible] good eating habits.

9

Diet for Boys and Girls

The period of transition from childhood to adulthood is called adolescence with accelerated physical, biochemical and emotional development. It is during this period that the final growth spurt occurs. There are many body changes which result due to the influence of hormones. The growth spurt of the boys are slower than that of the girls. The growth spurt signalling the onset of a critical body composition of 10 per cent body fat. However 22 per cent of body fat is required to maintain regular ovulation.

Greatest nutrient need for boys is between 12-15 years and for girls is 10-13 years. Both males and females are influenced by the adequacy of zinc status. They attain their adult stature between 18-20 but bone mass continues to increase upto age of 25. With the profound growth of adolescence there is increased demands for energy, protein, minerals and vitamins.

The dimensional changes and changes in maturational timing over the generations are called secular changes, the term secular referring to successive periods of time. Magnitude of secular trend in stature which may approximate 1 cm/decade and the inverse secular trend in menarcheal timing, which may approximately 0.2 yr/decade. Adolescent anorexia may lead to diminution of the secular trend.

The RDA of adolescents is given in Table.

Food Requirements

Energy : Caloric needs increase with the metabolic demands of growth and energy expenditure. Although individual needs vary, girls consume fewer kilo calories than boys. Boys need 2500-2600 kcal a day. Sometimes the large appetite characteristic of this growth period leads adolescents to satisfy their hunger with snack foods that are high in sugar and fat and low in protein. The calories for both boys and girls from the age group of 1-3 years to 7-9 years remain the same. During the adolescent year from the age of 10 years there is a marked difference in the caloric needs of boys and girls. As seen from the below the needs of boys are higher than those of girls.

Recommended Dietary Allowances of Adolescents

Nutrient	*Years*			
	13-15		*16-18*	
	boys	*girls*	*boys*	*girls*
Body weight kg	47.8	46.7	57.1	49.9
Energy kcal	2450	2060	2640	2060
Protein g	70	65	78	63
Fat g	22	22	22	22
Calcium mg	600	600	500	500
Iron mg	41	28	50	30
Vitamin A mcg	600	600	600	600
Beta carotene	2400	2400	2400	2400
Thiamine mg	1.2	1	1.3	1
Riboflavin mg	1.5	1.2	1.6	1.2
Niacin mg	16	14	17	14
Pyridoxin mg	2	2	2	2
Ascorbic acid mg	40	40	40	40
Folic acid mcg	100	100	100	100
Vitamin B_{12} mcg	0.2-1	0.2-1	0.2-1	0.2-1

Age in Years Comparison of energy RDA of different age groups

Proteins : For most adolescents, eating to satisfy appetite offers a reasonably sensitive indicator of energy needs. Protein needs represent 12-14 per cent of energy intake. The protein intake usually exceeds 1 g/kg body weight. This meets growth needs and for the pubertal changes in both sexes and for the developing muscle mass in boys.

The protein requirements for both boys and girls are the same up to the age of ten years. But there is a gradual difference in their requirements from the age of 10 years where the boys have a higher requirement compared to girls. This pattern is similar in calorie requirement.

Minerals : Calcium and iron are particularly needed during adolescence. Bone growth demands calcium. About 150 mg of calcium must be retained each day to allow for the increase in bone mass. Iron needed for haemoglobin synthesis necessitated by the considerable expansion of blood volume and for myoglobin needed for muscle growth. The girls need to ensure adequate intake of iron as they lose 0.5 mg/day by way of menstruation. The daily menstrual loss of iron is computed from the iron content of blood lost during the menstrual period averaged over a month. If this lost iron is not replaced, it predisposes to iron deficiency anaemia. During adolescence there is an increase in body mass corresponding to about 4.3 kg/year in the male and 4 kg/year in the female. With a further increase in haemoglobin by 2 g/dl in the male and 1 g/dl in the female, the respective requirement for growth alone is 0.7 mg/day in males and 0.45 mg/day in females while the obligatory losses also increase with age.

Vitamins : The need for thiamine riboflavin and niacin, increases directly with increased caloric intake. Folacin and B_{12} are essential for DNA and RNA synthesis and needed in higher amounts when tissue synthesis is occurring rapidly.

Tissue growth involves amino acid metabolism particularly transamination to synthesis non-essential amino acids. So the requirement for B_6 is increased. Premenstrual tension can be reduced if adolescent girls consume 100 mg/ day vitamin B_6. Skeletal growth requires vitamin D while the structural and functional integrity of newly formed cells depends on the availability of vitamins A, C and E.

Choice for Food

Physical and psychosocial pressures influence adolescents' eating habits. The boy fares better than the girl in that his large appetite and sheer volume of food leads him to consume adequate nutrients but the adolescent girl is less fortunate because (a) her physiologic sex differences associated with fat deposits during this period and comparative lack of physical activity she may gain weight easily, (b) social pressures and personal tensions concerning figure control will cause her to follow unwise, self-imposed crash diets for weight loss. (c) self starvation may result in complex and far reaching eating disorders like anorexia nervosa and bulimia.

Teenagers have the reputation of having the worst eating habits. They may skip a meal. Or they may east fast foods which are generally inadequate in calcium and vitamin A but high in calories, saturate fat and sodium.

Dietary Guidelines : Diet in adolescents is very significant because it influences the future nutritional status.

- Adequate well balanced nutritious foods should be taken to prevent obesity or undernutrition.
- An adolescent girl should take enough calcium rich foods in her diet to increase bone density which delays the onset of osteoporosis.
- No meal of the day should be missed.
- Avoid empty calorie foods such as carbonated beverages.
- Iron rich foods may be included in the diet to prevent anaemia.
- Calorie and protein rich foods should be taken to support the growth spurt.
- Include fruits and vegetables in the diet to meet the vitamins, minerals and fibre requirement.
- Eating habits should be independent of emotions.

Different Matters

Obesity : It affects 10-20 per cent of adolescent population. An excessive intake of kilocalories is less often the cause than lack of exercise. Concern about personal appearance may make the adolescent more reluctant to participate in activities like dance or sports that control weight. Other causes of obesity may be family habits, emotional stress and hormonal imbalance.

Eating Disorders : There are three recognised eating disorders—anorexia nervosa, bulimia nervosa and binge eating disorder.

Anorexia Nervosa

Physical Signs

- Onset in early to middle adolescence.
- Extremely thin or emaciated (less than 85% of normal or ideal body weight).
- Rapid loss of weight.
- Loss of menstrual periods.
- Development of lanugo, a fine, downy hair on arms, legs, and some times cheeks.
- Complaints of nausea, bloating, or constipation after eating normal amounts of food.

Food and Exercise Habits

- Cooking for others or obsessing about food but not eating.
- Rigidly avoiding specific foods or whole categories of food (dairy, meats, fats, etc.).
- Refusing to eat, denying hunger, eating tiny portions of food.
- Exercising excessively.
- Possessing in-depth knowledge of calories and fat in foods.
- Consuming odd food combinations or large amounts of low-calorie condiments (e.g., mustard, vinegars).
- Exhibiting ritualistic eating behaviors, such as cutting foods into tiny bits or using special utensils or plates each time when eating.
- Avoiding social invitations because of food that might be served.

Psychological Signs

- Feeling "fat" even when emaciated, intense fear of gaining weight, distorted body image.

- Excessive preoccupation with weight, food, exercise, and dieting.
- Social withdrawal, depression, moodiness.
- Emotional withdrawal.
- Perfectionism.
- Refusal to admit eating patterns are abnormal.
- Low self-esteem.
- Fatigue or weakness due to malnutrition.

Bulimia Nervosa

Physical Signs

- Onset in late teens or early twenties, often after weight loss or dieting attempts.
- Usually near ideal body weight, but often with weight fluctuations.
- Eats *very* large meals, but without gaining weight.
- Dental enamel erosion, cavities.
- Swollen cheeks (swollen parotid glands).
- Calluses on back of hands.
- Fatigue or weakness due to malnutrition.
- Irregular menstrual periods.

Food and Exercise Habits

- Frequent binge eating.
- Strict dieting followed by bingeing.
- Leaving room after eating, often to bathroom.
- Purging via diuretics, laxatives, emetics such as syrup of ipecac, or enemas, over-exercising, fasting, or vomiting.
- Hiding eating from others.
- Avoiding social invitations because of food that might be served.

Psychological Signs

- Excessive preoccupation with weight, food, exercise, and dieting.
- Feeling uncomfortable eating in front of others.

- Feeling out of control when eating and unable to stop binges.
- Depression, loneliness, shame, and feeling of emptiness (although may pretend to be cheerful).
- Alcohol or drug use, personal problems.
- Realization that eating patterns are abnormal.
- Low self-esteem.

Binge Eating Disorder

Physical Signs

- Onset at any age, often not recognized until adulthood.
- Usually overweight or obese.
- May have obesity-related diseases, such as type II diabetes, high blood pressure, high cholesterol.

Food and Exercise Habits

- Frequent dieting.
- Losing and regaining weight (weight cycling) or chronically dieting without losing weight.
- Frequent binge eating or eating when not hungry.
- Eating to point of extreme discomfort.
- Frequently eating large amounts in short time.
- Hiding eating or eating only small amounts when with others.
- Avoiding social invitations because of food that might be served.
- Having difficulty exercising because of excess weight.
- Trying to avoid physical activity or anything that might call attention to or increase own awareness of one's body.

Psychological Signs

- Depression, loneliness, shame, guilt, and emotional emptiness.
- Feeling out of control when eating and unable to stop binges.
- Eating to escape from emotions (anxiety, worry, or emotional pain).

- Feeling uncomfortable eating in front of others.
- Being preoccupied with food, dieting, body weight.
- Feeling irritable when withdrawing from binge or trying to diet, and depressed and sleepy immediately after overeating.
- Realizing that eating patterns are abnormal.
- Having low self-esteem.

Eating disorders are complex problems that are best treated by a team of health care specialists including medical, psychological and nutrition professionals.

Predisposition to Osteoporosis : Excessive exercise, high fibre, low fat intake lead to low circulating estrogen levels, irregular menses and low bone mass. Predisposition to osteoporosis is in part atleast is the result of dietary deficiency and exercise patterns during the developmental years. Low dietary intake of calcium rich foods such as milk in teenagers could be because of the misunderstanding about the amount of fat provided by the milk and substitution of milk with soft drinks. Bone density can be increased by including in the diet calcium rich foods.

Anaemia : There does seem to be a trend towards a decrease in the age at menarche over the decades both in the rural and urban situations, not only in the affluent upper classes but also among the poor classes of urban and rural communities and making adolescent girl susceptible to anaemia.

Anaemia is most common in all the groups of adolescent girls to the tune of 20-25 per cent irrespective of the social class. Angular stomatitis and glossitis are more common in poor classes because of the poor quality of diet.

Anaemia is common in poor class since intake is poor mainly due to the non-availability of healthy foods. In higher classes personal likes and dislikes and food taboos lead to anaemia. Supplementation of iron to mothers to be is the rational way to combat anaemia.

Undernutrition : Results of the studies conducted at National Institute of Nutrition Hyderabad (1990) showed a higher percentage of upper-middle class girls (36%) had deficit in BMI indicating that the weight deficit is a major factor, possibly related to the poor energy intake of this group of population. While among the urban poor and rural girls, this is mainly due to their getting lower priority for the food over the boys in the family. In the upper class, the weight deficit is related to the personal likes and dislikes and also a conscious attempt towards maintaining a low weight in the fear of becoming overweight.

Premenstrual Syndrome : This is not so uncommon in adolescence and is characterised by physical and psychological symptoms which occur 7-10 days prior to the onset of periods and disappear within the first day or two of menstrual flow. These include weight gain, abdominal bloating, breast engorgement and pain, constipation, peripheral oedema, headache, irritability, anxiety, depression, tension, fatigue, lack of concentration, increased appetite, craving for sweet and salty foods. The etiology and pathophysiology have not been identified. Management includes reassurance, exercise and dietary modifications to meet all the nutritional requirements.

Reason for Wrongs

Often a significant proportion of Indian girls get married soon after menarche and bear a child when she herself is still a child. These child-mothers are considered 'high risk' as maternal and perinatal death rates and infant mortality rates are higher among them. In India almost 40 per cent of girls are married at early age and have the first child before 18 years of age. Pregnancy is optimal when the mother is biologically mature. A biologically mature female is a young woman who is atleast 5 years post-menarchal and this has greater impact on pregnancy than her chronological age.

Nutritional deficiency signs get aggravated if the adolescent girl conceives immediately after menarche since she has to meet the demands of not only her growth, but also that of conceptus. This incidence of both preclampsia and eclampsia have been found to be higher and so also the incidence of pregnancy wastages.

In the poorer section of the society, complications are more common in adolescents, which have a direct bearing on the outcome of pregnancy.

Studies on age-related infant mortality in various parts of the country have shown that early neonatal deaths are almost double in the adolescent age group. Maternal mortality again is high due to eclampsia and haemorrhage.

There is a close association between the maternal body weight and the incidence of low birth weight. The lactation failure is also a more common occurrence among the adolescents, resulting in high infant mortality and morbidity due to earlier introduction of supplements. Due to small size of the pelvis, there is increase in the rate of premature deliveries and also high incidence of low birth.

Pregnancy and child birth are safest not at 15 but between 25 and 30 years.

Suggested Recipes during Adolescence

Recipe	*Reasons*
Samosa with channa, uthapam (cereal + pulse)	To meet increased needs of calories and protein.
Bajji, bonda, hamburgers Spring rolls, pizzas	Adolescents are fascinated by junk foods but one can select these. Rich in calories.
Basundi, ladoos	Protein rich foods meet growth needs.
Instead of carbonated cool drinks fresh juices can be given	Vitamin C requirement can be met.
Rice and rajmah, vegetable fried rice, pav bhaji omelette	Nutritious and give variety.

10

Diet for the Youth

Man needs a wide range of nutrients to perform various functions in the body and to lead a healthy life. During adulthood nutrients are required for the purpose of energy, for replacement of wornout tissues and maintenance of body functions. Though there is no growth during adulthood, protein is required for the replacement of wornout tissues. The nutritional requirement of other age groups is sometimes extrapolated from adults' requirements.

Food Requirements

Energy : Energy requirements of an adult man and woman are based on Reference man and Reference woman. Energy requirements for other individuals of different body weights and age are calculated.

Reference man is between 20-39 years of age and weighs 60 kg. He is free from disease and physically fit for active work. On each working day he is employed for 8 hours in occupation that usually involves moderate activity. While not at work he spends 8 hours in bed 4-6 hours sitting and moving around and 2 hours in walking and in active recreation or in household duties.

Recommended Dietary Allowances for an Adult Man and Woman

	Man			*Woman*		
Nutrient	*Sedentary*	*Moderate*	*Heavy*	*Sedentary*	*Moderate*	*Heavy*
Energy kcal	2425	2875	3800	1875	2225	2925
Protein g	60	60	60	50	50	50
Calcium mg	400	400	400	400	400	400
Iron mg.	28	28	28	30	30	30
Vitamin **A**						
Retinol mcg	**600**	**600**	**600**	**600**	**600**	**600**
Carotene mcg	**2400**	**2400**	**2400**	**2400**	**2400**	**2400**
Thiamine mg	**1.2**	**1.4**	**1.6**	**0.9**	**1.1**	**1.2**
Riboflavin mg	1.4	1.6	1.9	1.1	1.3	1.5
Niacin mg	16	18	21	12	14	16
Pyridoxin mg	2	2	2	2	2	2
Vitamin C mg	40	40	40	40	40	40
Folic acid mcg	100	100	100	100	100	100
Vitamin B_{12} mcg	1	1	1	1	1	1

Reference woman is between 20-39 years of age, healthy and weighs 50 kg. She may be engaged for 8 hours in general household work, in light industry or in other moderately active work. Apart from 8 hours in bed she spends 4-6 hours sitting or moving around in light activity and 2 hours in walking or in active recreation or in household duties.

An important factor which determines energy needs is the nature and duration of physical activity, whether moderate or heavy. For those whose occupation entails heavy work, allowances have to be higher than for those who are either, sedentary or engaged in moderate work. The allowances are made under the assumption that the energy expenditure for non-occupational activities remains unchanged. Table below gives ICMR RDA for an adult. The average calorie requirement for light, moderate and heavy activities are 225, 375 and 525 calories per hour respectively for an adult man. Excess energy in adults leads to undesirable consequences.

Protein : The average daily protein requirement of an Indian adult, in terms of a high quality protein like milk, egg at the physiological level is estimated to be 0.5 g/kg of body weight. One gram per kilogram of body weight is the RDA for men as well as women is suggested considering protein of mixed vegetable origin with NPU 65 relative to egg. The estimates of nitrogen losses and the amount of nitrogen needed to maintain balance have a co-efficient of variation in the same individual from day to day. The figure of 1.0 g/kg body weight includes a 30 per cent addition to cover this variability.

Protein/Calorie Ratio of Diets : It is useful to consider together the protein and energy requirement on habitual Indian diets. The protein requirement can be expressed as the ratio of protein calories to total dietary calories (PE %).

This concept is useful because in many population groups enough diet is not consumed to meet energy needs resulting in energy deficits. It will be seen that a PE% between 8 and 12 would meet the protein requirement of any group provided its energy needs are met.

Fat : In the diets of adults in India, about 20 per cent energy may be derived from fats. At all levels of calorie intake, invisible fat furnishes about 9 per cent energy and visible fat 10 per cent. This would come to 10-20 g. of fat per day depending upon the level of calories consumed. In habitual diets of our country, which are cereal-legume based, about half the invisible fat (6 per cent energy) is composed of linolic acid. The Expert FAO/WHO consultation committee has placed it at 3 per cent energy.

It has also been deduced to be 5g per day. This requirement can be met even by the invisible fat component of existing Indian diets. Saturated fatty acids, cis-monosaturated fatty acids, proteins and cholesterol can increase essential fatty acid requirement. It would appear prudent to choose the visible or cooking fat from unsaturated vegetable oils. Average Indian diet predominantly based on cereals and pulses including the diets of poor income groups, carry sufficient amount of linoleic acid.

Classification of Activities based on Occupation

	Male	*Female*
Sedentary	Teacher, tailor, barber, executive shoemaker, priest, retired personnel, landlord, peon, postman	Teacher, tailor executive, housewife
Moderate	Fisherman, basket maker, potter goldsmith, agricultural labour, carpenter, mason, rickshaw-puller, electrician, fitter, turner welder, industrial labour, coolie, weaver, driver	Servant, maid, coolie, basket-maker, agricultural labour, beedi-maker.
Heavy	Stone cutter, blacksmith, mine-worker, wood cutter, gangman	Stone cutter

Minerals : The requirement of calcium prescribed by ICMR is same for both men and women. To meet this requirement an adult needs to take atleast 200 ml. of buffaloe's milk or 350 ml of cow's milk. It is usually suggested that a C : P in the diet should remain somewhere between 1:1 and 1:2.

Iron requirement for woman is 2 mg. higher than man. Iron loss through menstruation in women of reproductive age groups are 0.6 mg./ day on an average, when spread over the whole month.

Vitamins : The requirement of vitamin A is same for both men and women. The requirement of B vitamins is based on calorie requirement (0.5 mg. of thiamine, 0.6 mg. of riboflavin and 6.6 mg of niacin per 1000 calories). Hence requirements of B vitamins are higher for moderate and heavy workers.

An intake of 20 mg of vitamin C may be sufficient to maintain the ascorbic acid levels in the adults. Taking into account that 50 per cent of vitamin C is lost in cooking, 40 mg is suggested for all adults. Where there is minimal exposure to sunlight, a specific recommendation of a daily supplement of 400 ug. of vitamin D is made. The requirement of vitamin E suggested is 0.8 mg/ g of essential fatty acids.

Balanced Diet

The overall production of food grains (cereals/millets/pulses) recorded a significant increase from about 108 million tonnes in 1970-71 to a little over 198 million tonnes during 1996. Though production of cereals and millets appears to be adequate, production of pulses, the most inexpensive source of protein for the rural poor, actually shows a decline. Total production of vegetables is about 30% less than the demand. The total production of milk is about 66 million tonnes, corresponding to about 197 g per capita per day which is much below the RDA of 250 g.

The distribution of foods, both within the community and the family, is unfavourable to some vulnerable groups due to low income and purchasing power, further reducing the availability of these foods. In view of the high cost of milk and flesh foods a large proportion of the Indian population subsists on diets consisting mostly of plant foods with low nutrient bio-availability. National Nutrition Monitoring Bureau surveys indicate that the daily intake of most foods in Indian households, except for cereals and millets (470 g) is much below the RDA. The diets provide negligible amounts of protective foods like pulses (29 g) and vegetables. Consumption of green leafy vegetables (< 10 g) and other vegetables (70-80 g) which are rich sources of micronutrients like beta carotene, folate, calcium, riboflavin and iron, is woefully inadequate. Intake of visible fat is less than 60% of the RDA.

The table below gives Nutritional and Health Status of Indians.

Nutritional and Health Status

	Prevalence (%)
Adults (%)	
Chronic Energy Deficiency (BMI < 18.5)	50
Anaemia in Pregnant women	70-90
General Population	
Anaemia (%)	50
Goitre (millions)	40
Cretinism (millions)	2.2
Still births due to IDD	90,000

Prevalence of Chronic Diseases

	Urban		*Rural*	
	Male	*Female*	*Male*	*Female*
Hypertension (%)	22.0	25.3	11.9	9.4
Obesity BMI (> 27) (%)	36.7	48.6	8.4	11.4
Diabetes Mellitus (%)	13.0	9.9	2.8	2.7
Coronary Heart Disease (%)	8.7	8.8	4.5	6.0
Cancer Incidence[b] (per million)	824	984	415	408

*< Mean- 2SD

a : ICMR Multicentric Study—Delhi (Urban); Haryana (Rural)—Unpublished.

b : National Cancer Registry Programme, ICMR, 1992.

Persistent under-nutrition throughout the growing phase of childhood leads to short stature in adults. About a half of the adults have a Body Mass Index below 18.5, which indicates chronic energy deficiency. It is estimated that nutritional anaemia contributes to about 85,000 maternal deaths every year and is one of the important causes of low birth weight. It adversely affects work output among adults.

On the other side of the spectrum of malnutrition, diet related non-communicable diseases are commonly seen. With increasing urbanisation, energy-rich diets containing higher amounts of fat and sugar, which also provide less dietary fibre and complex carbohydrates are being consumed, particularly in high-income groups. In addition, the urban population is tending to be more sedentary with little physical activity. Hence prevalence of disorders like obesity, heart disease, hypertension and diabetes is on the increase.

Sufficient Food

Diets of poor can be improved nutritionally by 1. replacing a single cereal with mixed cereals, one of them being a millet 2. inclusion of atleast 50 g. green leafy vegetables to improve the intake of vitamin A, iron and calcium 3. inclusion of inexpensive yellow fruits like papaya or mango and greens to increase vitamin A and C intake 4. inclusion of atleast 150 ml, of milk improves intakes of riboflavin, calcium besides improving protein quality of the diet. 5. Another extra 10 g of oil increases energy and essential fatty acid intake. An example of low cost improved diet by modifying the existing diet as suggested by ICMR is given in Table below.

Low Cost Balanced Diet for Sedentary Man

Ingredients	*Amount g.*
Cereals	460
Pulses	40
Leafy vegetables	50
Other vegetables	60
Roots and tubers	50
Milk	150
Oil and fat	40
Sugar and Jaggery	30

Reducing the Cost of a Meal

- Foodstuffs that are distributed through public distribution system (Ration shops) can be used.
- Inclusion of millets like ragi, jowar and bajra can reduce the cost of a meal.

- Cereals, since they are less expensive, can be increased to more than the normal amount present in a balanced diet.
- Unbranded foods can be included.
- Broken rice, broken eggs (fresh) left over vegetables and fruits (in the shop at the end of the day) cheaper cuts of meat can be bought.
- Greens particularly from trees like drumstick or agathi are cheaper and locally available or kitchen garden produce can be used.
- Fermenting, malting and sprouting can be done at home which enhance the nutritive value without increasing the processing cost.
- Inclusion of dry fish (like nethili) may supply good amount of nutrients without increasing the cost.
- Leaves of cauliflower, carrots, knol khol and beet root which are highly nutritious can become part of a meal. Curry leaves can also be used for better purpose in the diet.
- Recipes made at home are cheaper than bought. Home made food can be carried to the workplace instead of buying from the canteen.
- Steamed foods are less expensive than fried foods. Low cost diets have less amount of fats oil and sugars.
- Toned milk with low fat is less expensive but gives all the other nutrients except fat.
- Pulses like horse gram can be included to reduce the cost of a meal.
- Jaggery can be used instead of sugar.
- Inclusion of locally available ingredients and seasonal foods reduce the cost of a meal.
- Inexpensive and nutritious fruits like papaya and guava can be included in the diet.
- Low priced biscuits can be used as snacks in the diet.
- Natural foods are less expensive compared to processed and preserved foods.

11

Diet for the Aged

Old age is best defined as the age of retirement that is, 60 years and above. Improvement in health care technology has resulted in increased life expectancy. The number of persons in old age has increased. In India, the elderly constitute about 7 per cent of the total population and by 2016, the number is likely to increase to 10 per cent.

Prevailing Oldage

Ageing is a normal process begins at conception and ends only with death. Individuals are known to age at different rates. Heredity and good nutrition may slow the ageing processes so that the individual enjoys physical and mental vigour in his eighties. Goal of nutritional care should be to help the aged achieve a healthy, purposeful and independent living.

One prominent theory of ageing—the free radical theory—involves the continuous formation of free radicals as a result of exposure to oxygen and harmful exposure to environmental factors. These highly reactive substances lead to damage and alterations in the structure of proteins, lipids, carbohydrates and chromosomal material in cells which probably leads to changes associated with ageing.

Tissue damage by free radicals and pro-oxidant radicals like superoxide, peroxide and hydroxyl radicals is the basis for inflammatory and degenerative changes seen in variety of diseases like cancer. Endogenous anti-oxidants are superoxide dismutase (SOD) catalase (CAT) glutathione peroxidase (GPX) which act together with glutathione (GSH) and NADPH. With age and in diseases these antioxidant defenses are lowered and the vitamins A, C and E get excessively utilised and a deficiency state occurs.

The process of ageing brings about physiological, psychological and immunological changes which influences the nutritional status. The changes associated with ageing are partly influenced by genetics, race and gender.

As part of ageing process the functioning of the organ may change which may influence nutrient status as given in Table below

Food Requirements

These are based on the physiological changes that take place during old age. The nutritional requirements change after the age of 30 years.

Changes in organ function with ageing that may influence nutrient requirements

Organ or function	*Changes*	*Effect on nutrition*
Taste and smell	• Decreased taste buds and papillae on tongue. • Decrease in taste and olfactory nerve endings.	• Loss of ability to detect salt and sweet. • Decreased palatability causing poor food intake. • Decreased sensory stimulation that may impair metabolic processes.
Salivary glands	• Decrease in salivary secreation causes feeling of dry mouth, xerostomia.	• Difficulty in chewing and swallowing make them avoid certain foods particularly crunchy, dry and sticky foods.

Contd...

Organ or function	*Changes*	*Effect on nutrition*
Teeth	• Loss of teeth and wearing dentures.	• Decreased consumption of meats and fresh fruits and vegetables. In turn this can result in inadequate intake of energy, iron and vitamins particularly vitamin C, folate and beta carotene.
Gastric function and emptying	• Decreased secretion of hydrochloric acid, intrinsic factor and pepsin.	• Decreased bio-availability of minerals, vitamins and proteins.
	• > 60 years of age rapid rate of emptying of liquids.	• Decreased absorption of protein bound vitamin B_{12} and folate.
	• Increased proximal small bowel pH and bacterial overgrowth in bowel.	• Increase in bacterial folate synthesis to counteract malabsorption.
	• Decreased calcium absorption	• Poor vitamin D nutriture
Small intestine	• Decreased secretion of lactase.	• Can be a risk factor for developing osteoporosis.
	• Constipation—prolonged rectosigmoid transit.	
Liver and biliary function	• Decreased size and blood flow.	
	• Minor structural and biochemical changes.	• Rate of albumin synthesis may be decreased.
	• Gall bladder becomes sluggish in releasing bile.	• Susceptible to gallstones.
	• Activity of drug metabolising enzymes reduced.	• Drug dosages may need to be lower.
Metabolic function	• Impaired glucose tolerance.	• Requires dietary modifications, exercise and oral pharmacologic agents.
	• Decreased metabolic rate due to changes in body composition and reduction in physical activity.	• Requirement of energy decreases.
	• Body protein level decreases.	• Activity decreases.

Contd...

Organ or function	*Changes*	*Effect on nutrition*
Neurologic function	• Confusional states	• Decreased synthesis of serotonin, Carnitine derived from the amino acids lysine and methionine may be effective in slowing the mental deterioration in Alzheimer's disease. • Carotenoids seem to play a protective role related to ageing and cognitive function.
Immuno competence	• Declines with age	• Supplementation with vitamin E, zinc and poly unsaturated fatty acid can be increased.
Psychological factors	• Depression	• Can affect appetite, digestion, energy level, weight and well being.
Cardio vascular function	• Blood vessels become less elastic and total peripheral resistance increases.	• Prevalence of hypertension modification of diet accordingly.

Energy : After the age of 35 the basal metabolic rate decreases due to reduced muscle mass and other metabolically active tissue mass. Also there is reduction in physical activity which affects the energy needs.

The per cent muscle tissue decreases and fat tissue increases as the age increases. Resting metabolic rate decreases approximately 15-20 per cent over the life span, primarily due to changes in body composition and reduction in physical activity.

Sarcopenia, an age related loss in skeletal muscle is the result of a decline in muscle strength. Sarcopenia contributes to changes in gait and balance and loss of physical function. Lean body mass declines approximately 2 to 3 per cent per decade. Body protein level in the healthy elderly is 30-40 percent less than that in young adults.

The average body fat percentage in males increases from about

15 per cent when young to 25 per cent at the age of 60 years. This change in body fat is attributable to less intense physical activity and to an alteration in testosterone and growth hormone production that affects anabolism and lean tissue growth.

The calorie intake should be adjusted to maintain the body weight constant. In the case of obese the calorie intake should be adjusted to reduce the body weight gradually to about normal level.

Energy requirement decreases with age beyond 30 years. The adjustment factor given earlier by FAO/WHO/UNO is adopted for Indians are used for computing the energy requirements of different age periods. ICMR energy requirements of adults of different ages are given in Table below.

Energy Requirement at different Ages of Adult Males and Females with different Body Weights (Kcal/24 hr)

			Age	*30 + to 59 Activity*	*+ yrs*	*Age*	*60 + yrs. Activity*
Sex	*Body weights (Kg)*	*BMR*	*Sedentary*	*Moderate*	*Heavy*	*BMR*	*Sedentary*
Males	45	1325	2120	2518	3313	1040	1664
	50	1380	2208	2622	3450	1105	1768
	55	1435	2296	2727	3588	1170	1872
	60	1485	2376	2822	3713	1235	1976
	65	1540	2464	2926	3850	1295	2072
	70	1595	2552	3031	3988	1360	2176
	75	1650	2640	3135	4125	1425	2280
Females	40	1120	1792	2128	2800	0965	1544
	45	1160	1856	2204	2900	1015	1624
	50	1200	1920	2280	3000	1065	1704
	55	1240	1984	2356	3100	1115	1784
	60	1285	2056	2442	3213	1165	1864
	65	1325	2120	2518	3313	1215	1944
	70	1365	2184	2594	3413	1265	2024

Although the energy requirements decrease, the requirements for protein, vitamins and minerals do not diminish.

Protein : As people age there is a decrease in skeletal tissue mass. This results in decrease in store of protein provided by skeletal muscle and may be inadequate to meet the needs for protein synthesis. Hence the dietary protein intake is more important to meet essential needs.

A protein intake of 1.0g per kilogram, the normal adult requirement, is safe during old age. Since caloric requirements are decreased without the corresponding decrease in protein, the food should be protein rich compared to normal adult food. To meet this adequate quantities of protein foods such as milk and curd can be included.

Due to decreased appetite and poor digestion, old people are likely to consume less protein. The serum albumin level is the most reliable indicator of protein nutriture. Deficiency of protein results in oedema, anaemia and lowered resistance to infection. Infection, altered gastrointestinal function and metabolic changes caused by chronic disease can reduce the efficiency of dietary nitrogen utilisation and increased nitrogen excretion.

Of the total caloric intake 11-12 per cent should be from protein.

Carbohydrate : An impaired glucose tolerance in the elderly person can lead to hypoglycaemia, hyperglycaemia and type II diabetes mellitus. Insulin sensitivity can be enhanced by balanced energy intake, weight management and regular physical activity. Emphasis is placed on complex carbohydrates and controlling the intake of simple sugars. Whole grain cereals and pulses should be included in the diet.

It is necessary that atleast 50 per cent of calories are derived from carbohydrates.

Since caloric requirements are reduced, carbohydrates intake is also reduced.

Lipids : Emphasis should be placed on reducing the intake of saturated fat and choosing monounsaturated or poly unsaturated fat sources.

Minerals : Calcium needs during old age increases. Women over 50 years of age who are not receiving estrogens require more calcium as there is increased losses resulting in demineralisation of bone and osteoporosis. For women over fifty 1000 mg/day is recommended for the following reasons.

(a) Calcium is available only from a limited number of foods.

(b) To compensate age-related bone loss and to improve calcium balance.

(c) To decrease the prevalence of fractures and dental decay.

The physiology of calcium homeostasis in ageing men over 65 is similar to that of women with respect to the rate of bone loss. Calcium absorption efficiency decreases, vitamin D levels decline and hence men also require more calcium.

Milk is an important source of calcium for elderly as it is in the diet of the young. Wise provisions for calcium throughout life may go far in assuring an above average measure of health, an increase in vitality and perhaps in the lengthened prime of life. As caloric requirement decreases, total food consumption decreases, hence calcium supplements are essential.

The iron deficiency seen in the elderly is due to inadequate iron intake, blood loss due to chronic disease and/or reduced non-heame iron absorption secondary to achlorhydria of atrophic gastritis. Iron absorption per se does not appear to decline significantly with age. Vitamin C deficiency may also impair iron absorption.

Mild anaemia affects the health of old people due to less efficient circulation of blood. Iron intake should be adequate to prevent anaemia. Iron requirement can be same as adult man, 30 mg. If there is anaemia, supplemental iron can be given. Consumption of liver once or twice a week is effective in combating such a tendency. Particular emphasis may be placed upon the inclusion of those green leafy vegetables which are good source of iron like mayalu, cauliflower greens and agathi and whole grain or enriched breads and to certain iron rich dry fruits, and use of iron fortified salt.

There is no evidence that moderate sodium restriction will

delay or prevent the onset of cardiovascular disease. It is believed that great restriction of sodium should not be attempted except under the advice of a physician in the treatment of specific disease condition. Infact, moderate amounts of salt help to improve the palatability and thus the acceptability to the diet.

Some features of old age such as delayed wound healing, decreased taste sensitivity and anorexia are also findings associated with zinc deficiency. However, healthy elderly subjects have been shown to be in zinc balance despite an apparent low dietary intake. Older people who avoid flesh foods may be at increased risk of poor zinc status.

Vitamins : Elderly people are at risk for vitamin D deficiency due to decreased exposure to sunlight or decrease in renal mass. Prudent dietary supplementation with calcium and vitamin D improves bone density and may prevent fractures in a healthy elderly population.

Stress, smoking and some medications can increase vitamin C requirement. The antioxidant vitamins, such as vitamin E, carotenoids and vitamin C have been promoted as agents that enhance the health of the elderly. Vitamin C may be protective against cataract at an intake level of between 150 and 250 mg per day which is possible to achieve from dietary sources alone. Vitamin E has also been found to be a potent nutrient for reducing the decline in cellular immunity that occur in the elderly.

Requirements for the vitamin B_6 are increased in many elderly persons owing to atrophic gastritis which interferes with absorption. Alcoholic and liver dysfunction are additional risk factors for a deficiency of vitamin B_6. It has a significant role in immune function. Alcoholism is a risk factor for folate deficiency. Severe deficiency of folic acid in the elderly may result in anaemias and elevated serum homocysteine levels a risk factor for cardiac disease. Diets are often lacking in folate, so consumption of folate rich foods should be encouraged.

The usual causes of vitamin B_{12} deficiency are atrophic gastritis and bacterial overgrowth, which decrease absorption and can lead to pernicious anaemia.

Recent research has shown that increased serum levels of vitamins B_6 B_{12} and folate confer protection against elevated serum homocysteine an independent risk factor for cardiovascular disease, depression and certain neurologic deficits.

Although over nutrition is relatively uncommon in the healthy elderly population, a maintenance level multi vitamin and mineral supplement may enhance immunity and may cure latent nutritional deficiency states that may be the basis for common complaints of some individuals.

All vitamin requirements remain the same as the adult requirement.

Water : It is essential for the older person as it is for the younger individual. The kidney can function more adequately when there is sufficient fluid (1.5 litres) and hence to eliminate the waste solids. Water stimulates peristalsis and thus aids in combating constipation. Water can be consumed as such or in the form of butter milk, fruit juices, porridge and soups.

Some elderly individuals may have a fading sense of thirst and may go for long periods without fluid. Others avoid liquid for fear of incontinence. Dehydration can result in mental confusion, headaches and instability. Elderly should be advised to consume some fluid at regular intervals even if they are not thirsty.

Fibre : Fibre stimulates peristalsis. There is great enthusiasm to encourage the consumption of fibre containing food but any increase should be gradual otherwise bowel discomfort, distension and flatulence will result. While rough fibre, bran and mature vegetables are not advised for the aged, the fibre of tender vegetables, fruits will make easier the passage of the food mass down the intestinal tract.

Fibre also helps in reducing cholesterol which may reduce the incidence of atherosclerosis. Excess of fibre may reduce the absorption of iron and certain trace elements.

Choice for Food

In nearly 60-65 years of one's life habits, especially those pertaining to diet usually get moulded by factors like heredity, health, family, education, occupation and numerous other social

A summary of the dietary modifications required during old age and the reasons of it are given in Table.

Different Matters

The elderly are at a risk of poor nutrition due to economic pressures, poor dentition reduced mobility, depression loneliness, ageing tissues and inadequate food consumption.

Osteoporosis : It is a condition associated with a loss in bone density and bone mass and is primarily found in middle age and elderly women. Its major symptom is an increased vulnerability to bone fractures.

Modification of Diet during Old Age

Dietary Modification	*Reason*
Foods must be soft, easily chewable.	Problems of dentition, fallen teeth or dentures.
Foods should be easily digestible.	Decreased production of digestive enzymes.
Restricted fat in the diet, inclusion of PUFA.	Susceptible to heart disease.
Foods rich in fibre should be given. Coffee, tea and cola beverages should be restricted.	To prevent constipation and reduce cholesterol level. Also to prevent colon cancer. May result in insomnia due to over stimulation
Foods rich in calcium like milk should be given.	To compensate the bone loss and reduce the incidence of osteoporosis.
Green leafy vegetables can be given liberally.	Source of nutrients like carotene, calcium, iron, riboflavin, folic acid and vitamin C, besides supplying fibre. Rich in antioxidants.
Foods of the elderly should consist of familiar foods. New foods are difficult to accept.	Unfamiliar or changes in the food pattern may lead to psychological problems like depression
Clear soup at the beginning of meal.	Aids digestion.
Small and frequent meals instead of three heavy ones.	Favour more complete digestion and free from distress.
A glass of hot milk just before going to bed.	May induce sleep.
Heavy meal at noon and light evening meal.	Sleep is less likely to be disturbed.

Contd...

Dietary Modification	*Reason*
Too many sweets with lot of fats and sugar should be avoided.	Too much of sugar may cause fermentation, discomfort due to indigestion and cause tooth ache and may increase cholesterol level. May lead obesity.
Plenty of fiuid.	To prevent constipation and dehydration.

In young people in good health, the rate of calcium resorption equals that of bone formation. As people age, resorption begins to predominate over the bone formation, eventually resulting in osteoporosis. In osteoporosis the total amount of bone is reduced, but the remaining bone is of normal composition and quality.

Due to the reduction in number of cells, there is a decrease in thickness of the cortex, a thinning of the trabeculae and increased porosity of bone. As a result fractures occur with greater frequency. Common fracture sites include the vertebrae, femur and radius and often these occur in spite of little or no trauma. The rate of femoral fractures alone doubles for each decade after the age of 50.

The cause of osteoporosis may be age related changes such as decreased estrogen production associated with menopause. The decline in circulating 17-beta-estradiol is the predominant factor in the accelerated bone loss that begins after the menopause and continues for 6 to 8 years. Decreased intestinal absorption of calcium and production of vitamin D, reduced physical activity and increased parathyroid hormone secretion may also cause osteoporosis.

The post-menopaused women with osteoporosis generally begins to bend resulting in height loss. The compact bone mass in the vertebrae is responsible for humped backs characteristic of many elderly people. Dissolution of the jaw bone is another frequent symptom of osteoporosis. It is a major contributing factor in periodontal disease, resulting in premature loss of teeth.

Although ageing is one universal and unavoidable factor that brings a risk of osteoporosis many avoidable risk factors like sedentary life-style, emotional stress, inappropriate diet may contribute for osteoporosis.

It is sensible to encourage all old people and especially those with radiological evidence of osteoporosis, to be as physically active as possible. The more they are on their feet, less is the risk of pathological fractures of the femur and spine.

It is sensible for old people to take a diet with ample calcium that is to drink a glass of milk regularly. Some old people have a markedly reduced capacity to absorb calcium from the gut and in such patients therapeutic doses of calcium salt might be of ample benefit. Adequate protein along with calcium also helps in the formation of bone tissue.

The incidence of osteoporosis is low in India compared to western countries. Prevalence of osteoarthritis in women is steadily increasing with age and obesity.

A study to assess the incidence of osteoporotic fracture was conducted among women admitted to the hospital by National Institute of Nutrition (98-99). It was observed that over 55 per cent of women above the age of 40 years had osteoporotic fractures, which confirms the problem of early onset of osteoporosis particularly among low socio-economic groups.

Treatment : Calcitonin and oestrogen are prescribed for osteoporosis. Calcitonin inhibits the reabsorption of bone calcium into the blood but has only a relatively short lived beneficial effect of 1 to 2 years. Oestrogen therapy in post menopausal women has been shown to slow the rate of bone loss although it does not stimulate new bone formation. It is much more effective as a preventive measure begun immediately after menopause than as a treatment of osteoporosis that has already developed. In the longer term, oestrogen treatment, results in increased parathyroid hormone and 1,25 $(OH)_2$ D synthesis, which may explain the observed improvement in the intestinal absorption and renal reabsorption of calcium.

Plant-based estrogens or phytoestrogens are used as adjunctive therapy for alleviating the symptoms of menopause. Phytoestrogens are nonsteroidal estrogens of dietary origin. Phytoestrogens in soya (isoflavones) may reduce the incidence of hot flashes, one symptom of menopause. Soya isoflavones may also protect women against osteoporosis by the action of genistein, which has an effect similar to estrogen. It stimulates osteoblasts, the bone-forming cells.

The most effective preventive measures are, ensuring calcium intake in adequate amounts throughout life and adopting a life-style that involves regular exercise and avoiding the avoidable risk factors.

Obesity : Some of the elderly are obese because their consumption of calories has not decreased though there is steady decrease in calorie requirement. Sedentary life-style may also be a contributing factor. Obese are susceptible to diabetes and mortality rate may be higher.

Neurological Dysfunction : Problems of disorientation and a slowing of neurological functioning, both seen in the elderly, have been attributed to various nutrient factors. A lack of niacin has long been associated with the dementia and depression of pellagra, a deficiency of choline hampers the synthesis of the neurotrans-mitter acetyl choline. Deficiencies of vitamin B_6 and thiamine are associated with central nervous system problem.

Women who walk or exercise regularly are less likely to experience the memory loss and other declines in mental function that can come with ageing.

Anaemia : Anaemia, characterised by feelings of fatigue, anxiety, lack of energy and sleeplessness is a common result of inadequate iron. Iron inadequacy can be caused by low dietary intake, impaired absorption possibly resulting from lack of haemiron or vitamin C or blood loss. Treatment may involve using iron supplements together with a diet providing iron sources of high bio availability and vitamin C to enhance absorption.

Pernicious anaemia is seen chiefly in middle ages and elderly persons (women aged between 45-65) Plasma vitamin B_{12} is below 160 ng/1 while plasma folate is usually normal. Hydroxy cobalamin should be given in a dosage of 1,000 mcg. The diet should include animal foods like liver, egg yolk, shrimps and curd.

Reason for Wrongs

The important causes of malnutrition during old age are :

(1) poverty

(2) inability to move around easily

(3) cumulative effects of chronic diseases necessitating multiple medications

(4) social isolation and

(5) lack of knowledge for adequate preparation of meals. Malnutrition is common among old people who are institutionalised.

Constipation : It is the infrequent passage of stools which are most often drier or harder than normal. Generally, it is uncomfortable and elimination can be difficult and painful. Common symptoms of constipation include bloating, sluggishness, a feeling of "fullness" in the rectum and a general sense of "feeling out of sorts".

The stools become hard and dry because the stool moves too slowly through the colon. The natural contractions or rhythms of the colon might be disturbed due to loss of tone, stress, medication, illness, resisting the urge to defecate, pain from haemorrhoids or tissues, lack of exercise, a low fibre diet or not drinking enough fluids. It may even be caused by overuse of stimulant laxatives or enemas.

Constipation can be prevented by eating regular meals, drinking plenty of fluids and doing exercise daily. One should respond to the urge to move bowels and avoid straining. And by adding fibre to the diet, constipation can be prevented.

Degenerative Diseases : Oxidative stress is able to promote the process of ageing and also able to increase the probability of age specific disease like atherosclerosis and cancer where free radicals are implicated. The incidence of cancer increases progressively with age. Resistance to disease declines in the elderly people.

Vitamin E retards coronary artery diseases. Diabetes mellitus in which vitamin C metabolism plays important role prevents complications. Persons with high antioxidant intake are less likely to develop certain cancers. Ocular diseases in which beta carotene is thought to decrease the risk of developing advanced or exudative age related macular degeneration. Antioxidants, vitamin C, E and beta carotene, thought, to be protective largely because they can inactivate free radicals which would otherwise damage the cells. Three daily servings of vegetables and two of fruits are recommended to fulfil these antioxidant vitamin requirement. The normal requirement of antioxidants without side effects are given Table below.

Requirement of Antioxidants

Nutrient	*Amount*
Vitamin E IU	100-3200
Vitamin C mg	500-1000
Carotenoids mg	10-50
Selenium mg	100-300
Zinc mg	15-25

Until more evidence is available it is prudent to advise intake of 600 g/ day of antioxidant rich food.

Diseases like diabetes, atherosclerosis, hypertension and cancer and disability disorders like bone fractures, arthritis and strokes may affect nutrient requirements, intake, digestion, absorption, metabolism and excretion.

If the damage from free radicals occurs within the collagen fibrous network underlying the skin, one may notice a sagging of the tissue, the appearance of fine lines and wrinkles and discolouration of the pigment. What we often assume are simply the visible signs of normal ageing are often the premature effects of excessive oxidative damage. This can be slowed down or even halted through nutrition supplements. Antioxidants, toss the electron hungry molecules (free radicals) and keeping them from damaging the body's cells. Antioxidants should be given to prevent degenerative diseases.

The elderly are more prone to diseases due to lowered food intake, physical activity and resistance to infection. The elderly need more calcium, iron, zinc, vitamin A and antioxidants to prevent age related diseases. Good food habits and regular exercise minimise the ill-effects of ageing.

Problems on Way

Clinical and biochemical investigations conducted by Natrajan, V.S. et al (Natrajan, V.S., 1991, *Nutrition in health and diseases in the elderly,* Government General Hospital Madras) have shown that fatigue, alteration in appetite, alteration in weight, shortness of breath and giddiness and joint pains are the common complaints during old age. Fatigue may be due to coexisting diseases like diabetes or ischemic heart diseases or due to pulmonary tuberculosis. Blunting of taste sensation may be due to degenerative changes in the parietal lobe of brain in old age. Loss of weight during old age may be due to consumption of less calories. Hypertension, diabetes and anaemia may be the cause of giddiness.

Drug-nutrient Reaction : The aged people constitute only 10 per cent of the total population but they consume about 25 per cent of drugs prescribed because of increased health problems in old age.

At any age there is a risk of harmful drug or drug nutrient interactions, but elderly persons seem to have more than their share. Several things contribute to this increased risk among the elderly.

1. They are likely to take more drugs for longer periods to control chronic diseases.
2. Illness, mental confusion or lack of drug information may increase errors in self-care.

Nutrients can affect drug action by altering the digestion, absorption, distribution metabolism and/or excretion of the drug. Drugs may exhibit their effects on nutritional status through several avenues effects on food intake, alteration of nutrient absorption, alteration of nutrient metabolism and alteration in nutrient excretion.

Because the rate of drug metabolism and detoxification in the liver is much slower in older people, drugs remain in the body longer to exert their influence on the metabolism of nutrients.

Effects of drugs on food intake and drug-induced vitamin effect are shown in Tables below.

Effects of Drugs on Food Intake

Drug	*Its effect*
I. Increased appetite	
1. Antihistamines (cypropheptadine hydrochloride)	Increase in appetite and subsequent weight gain.
2. Psychltropic drugs Chlordiazepoxide hydrochlo ride, diaxepam, Chloropromazine, hydrochloride	Hyperphagia (Tranquilisers may cause hypophagia in geriatric patients)
3. Steroids	Nitrogent retention, increased lean body mass and weight gain.
II. Decreased appetite	
1. Amphetamines	Depress the appetite and loss of weight.
2. Insulin	Insulin induced hypoglycaemia may cause nausea, weakness and aversion to foods.
3. Alcohol	Anorexia, reduced food intake and malnutrition.
III. Taste sensitivity	
Chelating agent D-penicillamine used in metal poisoning, rheumatoid arthritis or cystinuria.	Loss of taste (dysgensia) caused by zinc heavy deficiency.

Contd...

Drug	*Its effect*
Diuretics, anticancer agents such as methotrexate and agents used to treat Parkinson's disease Antibiotics, ampicillin, griseofulvin, streptomycin, anticoagulant, antihistamine, antihypertensive agents, anti-infectious agent (metronidazole) cholesterol lowering agent (clofibrate), hypoglycaemic agent, sodium lauryl sulphate of tooth paste	Loss of taste, smell can lead to overeating or may stop from eating.
IV. Nausea	
Cardiac glycosides digitals, drugs used in cancer chemotherapy	Nausea and vomiting Malnutrition and weight loss.
Bulking effects, Methyl cellulose	Decrease the intake of food may interfere with absorption of nutrients.
Increased absorption Cimetidine	Reduces gastric acid and volume output, improves absorption of protein and carbohydrate.
Decreased absorption colchicine (used in the treatment of gout)	Causes B_{12} deficiency
Alcohol abuse	Malabsorption of thiamine and folic acid.
Laxatives	Osteomalacia

Drug Nutritional Interactions

	Drug	Increased requirement	Potential mechanism	Deficiency symptoms
1	Antacids (aluminium and magnesium hydroxides)	Phosphate	Formation of insoluble salts	Malaise, paresthesias, anorexia.
2	Anticonvulsant (phenobarbital, phenytoin)	Vitamin D	Induction of hepatic microsomalenzymes resulting in inactive vitamin D metabolites.	Rickels, osteomalacia.
3	Oral contraceptives (norethind/one/ mestranol)	Folic acid	Inhibition of poly-glutamic folate absorption	Megaloblastic anaemia
4	Antituberculosis drugs (isoniazid cycloserine)	Vitamin B_6	Excretion of pyridoxal hydraxone complex	Peripheral neuropathy
5	Diuretics (benzothiadiaz ides)	Potassium	Enhancement of renal excretion	Hypokalaemia
6	Anticoagulants (coumarin)	Vitamin K	Inhibition of vitamin K recycling	Hypoprothrombi-nemia

Dietary Guidelines

- Empty calorie foods should be taken minimum and calorie dense foods should be avoided.
- Foods rich in protein vitamin and mineral should be included.
- Vegetables and fruits are good sources of antioxidants. A minimum of five servings should be taken.
- Fat promotes weight gain. Fat particularly saturated fat should be limited.
- Gas forming foods like sulphur containing vegetables and certain type of pulses have to be avoided.
- Soft well cooked foods are preferred.
- Fried and concentrated foods be avoided.
- Caffeine containing beverages should be limited otherwise may suffer from insomnia.
- High fibre diet including greens and whole grains are to be included in the diet.
- Easily digestable steamed foods like idlis, idiappam can be part of the diet.
- Plenty of fluids and semisolid foods should be taken.
- Excess salt intake should be avoided.
- 2-3 servings of low fat milk should be included in the diet.
- Tobacco chewing smoking and betel leaves chewing are the habits which may affect consumption of food in the elderly.

Studies have proved that those who walk or exercise regularly are less likely to experience the memory loss and other declines in mental function that can come with ageing. Exercise is an integral part of maintaining healthy life. It helps to regulate body weight. The risk of degenerative disease is considerably decreased by regular exercise.

First of October is Celebrated as 'World Elders Day'
Suggested Recipes during Old Age

Recipe	*Reason*
Pongal, idli, idiappam	Cereal pulse combination easily chewable and digested.
Tomato soup, rasam	Good appetiser, low calorific value aid in digestion.
Amarnath dal	Greens good sources of vitamins, minerals and fibre.
Buttermilk, fruit juices	As they are light old people may feel comfortable.
Banana	Prevents constipation.
Skimmed milk powder	High in protein and low in fat. The requirement of protein.
	Remains the same where is calorie intake is reduced.
Warm milk	Induces sleep.

12

Care for Mothers to Be

Adequate nutrition before and during pregnancy has greater potential for a long term health impact than it does at any other time. Maternal health is a complex, influenced by various genetic, social and economic factors, infections and environmental conditions, many of which may affect the foetal growth. Physiological adaptations result in improved utilisation of nutrients either through increased absorption, decreased excretion or alternations in metabolism.

A woman who has been well nourished before conception begins her pregnancy with reserves of several nutrients so that the needs of the growing foetus can be met without affecting her health. Infants who are well nourished in the womb, have an enhanced chance of entering life in good physical and mental health. The effects of undernutrition during reproduction will vary depending upon the nutrients involved, the length of time it is lacking and the stage of gestation at which it occurs.

A woman whose diet is adequate before pregnancy is usually able to bear a full term viable infant, without extensive modifications of her diet. Mother's diet should produce adequate nutrients so that maternal stores do not get depleted and produce sufficient milk to nourish her child after birth. The nutritional demands are highly increased in an adolescent mother.

Physical Aspects

Blood volume expands by 50% resulting in a decrease in haemoglobin levels, blood glucose values and serum levels of albumin, other serum proteins and water-soluble vitamins. The decline in serum albumin levels contributes to a tendency for extra-cellular water to accumulate during pregnancy. The decrease in water soluble vitamin concentration makes determination of an inadequate intake or a deficient nutrient state difficult. By contrast, serum concentrations of fat soluble vitamins and other lipid fractions, such as triglycerides, cholesterol and free fatty acids increase.

There is a decreased ability to taste saltiness. This may infact, be a physiologic mechanism for increasing salt intake. Increased progesterone level relaxes the uterine muscle to allow expansion with fetal growth. Gastrointestinal mobility diminishes, to allow for increased absorption of nutrients. This often results in constipation. Additionally, a relaxed lower oesophageal sphincter can cause regurgitation and heart burns.

Increased blood volume produces a high glomerular filtration rate. It appears that the renal tubules are unable to adjust completely and a percentage of nutrients that would have been reabsorbed in the non-pregnant women are excreted in the urine. Increased amounts of amino acids, glucose and water soluble vitamins may appear in the urine. This may be a reason for the increased number of urinary tract infections seen in pregnant women.

The ability to excrete water is lowered and oedema in the legs and ankles is common and normal.

Less than half of the total weight gain resides in the fetus, placenta and amniotic fluid; the remainder is found in maternal reproductive tissues, fluid, blood and maternal stores, a component composed largely of body fat. Gradually increasing subcutaneous fat in the abdomen, back and upper thigh serves as an energy reserve for pregnancy and lactation.

Increased weight gain during pregnancy is associated with

increased birth weight and a progressive decrease in the number of LBW infants.

Role of Placenta : The placenta is the principal site of production for several hormones responsible for regulation of fetal growth and development of maternal support tissues. It is also involved for exchange of nutrients, oxygen and waste products. Any derange to or inadequacy in the placenta compromises its ability to nourish the fetus, regardless of how well nourished the mother is or how optimal her dietary intake.

Preconceptual Nutrition : Maternal nutrition plays a role in certain types of fetal malformations or spontaneous abortion. Because these abnormalities occur so early in pregnancy (during organogenesis) modifications must be made before pregnancy begins. In diabetes, incidence of congenital defects can be reduced almost to normal by bringing the blood glucose under good control prior to pregnancy. Administration of folic acid 400-800 mcg per day around and during conception and early gestation can reduce the incidence of neural tube defects. In addition, women with low body weight and poor nutritional status prior to pregnancy have more low birth weight infants, premature spontaneous rupture of membranes, infection and anaemia.

On the other end of the spectrum, overweight women are more likely to have fetal death, diabetes, hypertensive disorders and labour abnormalities. Because these maladies are difficult to correct once pregnancy begins, a woman should achieve a body mass within 90-120% of ideal weight prior to conception.

Major Prenatal Nutrition Alterations

Haematologic staus

White blood cells

Serun albumin

Serum vitamin C, Folic acid and B_{12}

Serum carotene

Vitamin A

Serum tocopherol

Urinary N′-methylnicotinamide

Urinary riboflavin

Urinary xanthuric-acid excretion

Due to undernourishment of the mother the baby is at an increased risk of being premature with low birth weight and developmental irregularities. Intrauterine nutrition is highly important for the growth of the central nervous system and kidneys of the foetus which mature during the latter part of pregnancy. Therefore nutrition deficits before birth can never be wholly reversed after birth.

Schematic diagram, below shows the relationship between maternal and foetal nutrition.

Inadequate food intake and poor nutrient utilisation

↓

Maternal malnutrition

↓

Reduced blood volume expansion

↓

Inadequate increase in cardia output

↓

Decreased blood and nutrient supply to the foetus

↓

Reduced placental size

↓

Reduced nutrient transfer

↓

Foetal growth retardation

Fig. Relationship between maternal and foetal nutrition

Nutritional Requirements : Increase in nutritional requirements depend on the nature of metabolic changes of pregnancy and the nutrition reserves of the mother. The RDA of the expectant mother is given in Table below.

Recommended Dietary Allowances of an Expectant Mother

Nutrient	*Normal adult woman*	*Pregnant woman*
Energy kcals		
Sedentary	1875	+300
Moderate	2225	+300
Heavy	2925	+300
Protein g	50	+15
Fat g	20	30
Calcium mg	400	1000
Iron mg	30	38
Retinol mcg	600	600
Beta carotene mcg	2400	2400
Thiamine mg		
Sedentary	0.9	+0.2
Moderate	1.1	+0.2
Heavy	1.2	+0.2
Roboflavin mg		
Sedentary	1.1	+0.2
Moderate	1.3	+0.2
Heavy	1.5	+0.2
Niacin mg		
Sedentary	12	+2
Moderate	14	+2
Heavy	16	+2
Pyridoxine mg	2.0	2.5
Ascorbic acid mg	40	40
Folic acid mcg	100	400
Vitamin B_{12} mcg	1	1

Energy : Energy needs during pregnancy increase because of the additional energy required for the following.

- — The growth and physical activity of the foetus.
- — The growth of the placenta.
- — The normal increase in maternal body size.
- — The additional work involved in carrying the weight of the foetus and extra maternal tissues.
- — The slow but steady rise in basal metabolic rate during pregnancy. Any decrease in the activity of the mother decreases the caloric requirement.

For an Indian woman of 55 kg, the total energy cost of pregnancy is about 80,000 kcals. Of this about 36,000 kcals is deposited as fat which is utilised subsequently during lactation.

Hence ICMR recommended energy requirement of pregnant woman as follows:

Sedentary worker	1875 + 300 = 2175
Moderate worker	2225 + 300 = 2525
Heavy worker	2925 + 300 = 3225

The caloric requirements of a pregnant woman is mostly increased in the latter half of pregnancy.

The increase in calories for trimesterwise is as follows:

1st trimester	-	10 cals/day
2nd trimester	-	90 cals/day
3rd trimester	-	200 cals/day

Any decrease in the activity of the mother decreases the caloric requirement. It is very evident that normal pregnancy calls for a considerable weight gain over and above that represented by the size of the foetus. The fat that accumulates throughout pregnancy (specially for the first 30 weeks) acts as an energy reserve. When the supply of calories are inadequate the fat may be used up to provide the high energy needs of the rapidly growing foetus and to spare the proteins for tissue growth. This results in an increase in the ketones in the urine during the 1st trimester of pregnancy.

The foetus does not accumulate any fat except in the cell walls and system. All the fat is synthesised from glucose except for the only essential fatty acid (linoleic acid) which is transferred from the mother to the child.

Protein : The normal protein requirement of an adult woman is 50 g/day. ICMR increased the requirement during to 65 g/day. Additional protein is essential for:

1. Rapid growth of the foetus.
2. The enlargement of the uterus, mammary glands and placenta.
3. Increase in maternal circulating blood volume and subsequent demand of increased plasma protein to maintain colloidal osmotic pressure and circulation of tissue fluids.
4. Formation of amniotic fluid and storage reserves for labour, delivery and lactation.
5. The transfer of amino acids from the mother to foetus (upto 20 weeks all amino acids must be provided to the foetus as it cannot oxidise amino acids as a source of energy).

Protein requirement during pregnancy has been computed on the basis of N accretion. Based on the body weight gain of 12 kg in a normal healthy well nourished pregnant woman, the daily N deposited during the three trimesters is estimated to be 0.1, 0.5 and 0.9 g respectively. After increasing by 50 per cent to convert the factorial value into physiological value for N accretion, and 25 per cent for individual variation, the safe level of intake in terms of a high quality protein during the three trimesters will be 1.2, 6.0, 10.5 g respectively. After adjusting for the dietary protein quality of NPU 65, the safe intake during the latter half of pregnancy recommended by the Nutrition Expert Committee is 15g/day.

If protein requirements are not met during pregnancy:

1. There is increased risk of pregnancy.
2. The foetus may grow at the expense of mother.
3. Maximum growth of the baby cannot be obtained.
4. Number of cells in tissues particularly in brain may be less.

Protein and calorie deficiency during gestation may result in poor utilisation of food by off spring after birth and a failure to ever compensate for early food deprivation. When amino acids are transferred, some big protein molecules also cross the placental barrier which give immunity to the infants. In the total weight gain during pregnancy there is 1 kg of protein 1/2 of which is foetal tissue.

Milk, meat, egg and cheese are complete proteins and of high biological value. Additional protein may be obtained from legumes and whole grains, nuts and oil seeds.

Linoleic Acid : The requirements of linoleic acid during pregnancy is 4-4.5 en%. If invisible fat is 12.5 en% to meet, EFA, visible fat will be 30g/day.

Calcium : ICMR calcium requirement of adult woman is 400 mg/day. Requirement increases during pregnancy to 1000 mg/ day.

Although the infant bones are poorly calcified at the time of birth an appreciable amount of calcium is involved in foetal development. A full term foetal body is made up of 30 g of calcium.

Increased intake of calcium by the mother is highly essential, not only for the calcification of foetal bones and teeth but also for protection of calcium resources of the mother to meet the high demands during lactation.

Two-thirds of foetal calcium is transferred from the mother to the foetus after 30th week of pregnancy at the rate of 300 mg per day. Radio isotopic studies revealed that nearly 80 per cent calcium of the foetal skeleton and mother were obtained from the mother's diet, and the rest was obtained from maternal reserves. Pregnant woman usually absorb not less than 40 per cent of the calcium available in their diet. Calcium retention by pregnant woman is of 2 to 5 times the amount needed by the foetus in the 6th and 7th months of pregnancy indicating that maternal reserves are being built up at this stage. The amount of dietary calcium needed is reduced when vitamin D is available. Use of vitamin D and calcium reduces muscular cramps of pregnancy.

To prevent 'osteomalacia' mother's diet should contain less of phytic acid, adequate amounts of vitamin D and sufficient amount of calcium. Mothers should avoid repeated pregnancies.

Dairy products are a primary source of calcium. Green leafy vegetables also contribute to calcium.

Iron : Normal iron requirement of an adult woman is 30 mg/ day. ICMR requirements during pregnancy is 38 mg/day. The increase in iron by 8 mg/day can be attributed to the following:

- Infants are generally born with high Hb levels of 18-22 g/ 100 ml. of blood. Iron stores in the liver of the infant lasts from 3 to 6 months. Iron is also required for growth of foetus and placenta. To achieve these levels mother must transfer 240 mg of iron to the foetus during gestation.
- It is also required for the formation of haemoglobin as there is 40-50 per cent increased maternal blood volume. For this 400 mg of iron is required.
- Loss of maternal iron through skin and sweat is about 170 mg of iron. The total iron requirement for the entire period of pregnancy is 810 mg. The actual increase in requirement of iron is only in second and third trimester. But a single large dose of iron at the beginning of pregnancy is an effective way to build up iron stores and to protect against depletion of reserves. To avoid iron deficiency a woman should enter pregnancy with a store of atleast 300 mg of iron.

Liver, dried beans, dried fruits, green leafy vegetables, eggs, enriched cereals and iron fortified salt provide additional sources of iron.

Sodium : Normal adult woman's requirement of sodium should be maintained to prevent any defective disorders and deficiency.

1. During pregnancy there is an increase in the extra cellular fluid which calls for an 80 per cent increase in the body sodium. Restriction in the diet can cause a severe hormonal and biochemical changes.
2. When blood sodium level drops, kidney produces the hormone renin, as a result of which the sodium that is needed for use by the body is retained.

3. When the system is over taxed it can result in sodium deficiency causing an increased risk of eclampsia, prematurity and low birth weight of infants.

Uses of diuretics should be discouraged during pregnancy as they can cause loss of sodium.

Sodium is restricted when there is oedema or hypertension.

Iodine : Normal requirements are insufficient during pregnancy specially if mothers belong to the adolescent group. If increased demands are not met it may even result in onset of goitre. Iodine deficiency may also result from increased urinary loss. If mother has goitre, then the infant's chances of getting goitre increase by 10 times. Also the incidence of cretinism increases. Iodised salt can be used as a preventive measure. Iodine deficiency increases the risk of still birth and miscarriage.

Zinc : Zinc deficiency during the antenatal period leads to adverse effects on the newborn including foetal mortality, foetal malformations including -CNS teratogenecity and reduced intra uterine growth rate. Low zinc during pregnancy doubles the risk of low birth weight and trebles the risk of preterm delivery.

Vitamin A : Normal requirements of β-carotene for an adult woman is 2400 mcg. Same level is suggested during pregnancy. Vitamin A requirements during pregnancy have been calculated on the basis of the vitamin content of livers of the newborn. Additional intake of vitamin A required for this purpose is about 25 ug/day throughout pregnancy. Since this constitutes a small fraction of the recommended allowance for normal women, no additional dietary allowance during pregnancy is suggested. Liver, egg yolk, butter, dark green and yellow vegetables and fruits are good source of Vitamin A.

According to studies conducted at National Institute of Nutrition, Hyderabad (1985) that pregnant women of the low income groups have poor vitamin A status as judged by serum vitamin A levels. A daily supplementation of 6000 I.U. for about 12 weeks appears to improve serum vitamin A levels and correct vitamin A deficiency in these pregnant women. Improving vitamin A status of pregnant women reduces maternal mortality.

Excess vitamin A should not be taken during pregnancy.

Vitamin D : Vitamin D is highly essential as it enhances the maternal calcium absorption. Its active form calcidiol and calcitriol cross the placenta with ease and play an important role in calcium metabolism of the foetus. Maternal deficiency of vitamin D results in neonatal hypocalcaemia and hypoplasia. Excessive vitamin D can also result in complications such as atherosclerosis, hypercalcaemia, calcium deposits in various vital organs and mental retardation in the infants.

Vitamin E : In animals vitamin E has an important role to play in the reproductive process and reduces the number of spontaneous abortions and still births. In women it has not been evidently proved that vitamin E deficiency can cause pregnancy failure although they may prove beneficial to those who have had repeated spontaneous abortion or failure to conceive. Very little vitamin E crosses the placenta, so infant has low tissue concentrations that persist upto atleast 6 years. Requirement of vitamin E increases with increased intake of PUFA.

Vitamin K : Vitamin K is essential for synthesis of prothrombin that is necessary for normal coagulation of blood. It is highly essential for preventing neonatal haemorrhage. An oral dosage of menadione (synthetic form of vitamin K) during the last weeks of pregnancy or an injection during labour is essential to stimulate prothrombin synthesis. But care should be taken to see that the dosage is given at average level to prevent adverse effects.

Water Soluble Vitamins : Because little of water soluble vitamins are stored, the pregnant woman must rely on her daily intakes that is high enough to meet the added requirements of pregnancy. Generally maternal blood levels for water soluble vitamins tend to fall and foetal blood levels tend to exceed those of mother by 50 to 100 per cent during pregnancy.

Thiamin : ICMR recommendations of thiamin RDA for an adult woman is :

0.9 mg for sedentary worker

1.1 mg for moderate worker

1.2 mg for heavy worker

For a pregnant woman the requirement is increased by 0.2 mg/day.

The relationship between thiamin and caloric intake remains the same during pregnancy i.e., for 1000 calories 0.5 mg of thiamin are required. The normal urinary excretion of thiamine drops indicating that more is being retained and used by tissues. In some cases thiamin helps to relieve the nausea of pregnancy.

Riboflavin

ICMR recommendations of riboflavin RDA for an adult woman is :

1.1 mg for sedentary worker

1.3 mg for moderate worker

1.5 mg for heavy worker

In a pregnant woman the RDA is increased by 0.2 mg/day.

Requirements are increased due to increase in maternal body size and growth of foetus and accessory tissues. Riboflavin is present in higher amounts in the foetal blood than in maternal blood. Animal studies have shown that the lack of riboflavin interfere with cartilage formation resulting in skeletal malformations such as shortening of long bones and fusion of ribs.

Niacin

ICMR recommendations of niacin RDA for an adult woman is 12 mg for sedentary worker, 14 mg for moderate worker and 16 mg, for heavy worker. In a pregnant woman the RDA is increased by 2 mg, corresponding to the increase in calories. The conversion of amino acid into niacin is more efficient during pregnancy.

Vitamin B_6

Normal requirement of pyridoxine in an adult woman is 2.0 mg ICMR increased during pregnancy to 2.5 mg/day. During pregnancy due to normal stress the tryptophan metabolism is altered, resulting in decreased ability to convert tryptophan to niacin and this affects the cell growth. During "toxaemia of pregnancy". (high B.P., oedema, proteinuria) the B_6 levels are lower. Women who used oral contraceptives prior to conception often enter pregnancy with low tissue levels of vitamin B_6. There is no satisfactory theory to explain that these low levels affect the outcome of pregnancy but they do reduce the amount of pyridoxine in breast milk during lactation. B_6 is said to be used to control nausea of pregnancy.

Folic Acid

Normal adult woman requirement of folic acid is 100 mcg/ day. ICMR recommendations during pregnancy are 400 mcg/day. The recommended intake of folacin is based on its role in promoting normal foetal growth and preventing macrocytic anaemia of pregnancy. Iron deficiency puts additional stress on folate metabolism and may convert a sub clinical folate deficiency into megaloblastic anaemia. Folic acid is needed for the synthesis of essential components of DNA and RNA which increase rapidly during growth thereby increasing the requirements. Also folacin is essential for the development of RBCs which must increase as the mothers blood volume increases.

Once folate enters the foetal circulation it cannot be retransferred back into the maternal blood. There is notable decrease in folate absorption and an increase in urinary excretion during pregnancy which may contribute to maternal store depletion. Aminopterin, a folacin antagonist induces resorption of foetuses in animals. Its use in human beings leads to congenital malformation such as hare lip, cleft palate or hydrocephalus and complications of pregnancy "Abrupto placenta" i.e. premature detachment of the placenta, foetal malformation, haemorrhage which have all been identified as results of folic acid deficiency and cannot be supplemented after the onset of the problems. Thus folic acid deficiency is a major cause of concern in pregnancy and pregnancy is a major cause of folacin deficiency.

Supplementation of folic acid before conception and during the first 12 weeks of pregnancy is advisable to reduce the primary and secondary risk of neural tube defects—spina bifida and anencephaly in the foetus. Birth weights of infants born to mothers who had received 300 *ug* folate a day during pregnancy were higher than those born to mothers who had received either 100 or 200 *ug* daily. These findings suggest that pregnant women need 300 *ug* of additional folic acid daily.

Vitamin B_{12}

Normal adult woman's requirement of vitamin B_{12} is 1 mcg and this requirement remains the same even during pregnancy. The foetus has priority over the mother in B_{12}, and foetal blood had twice the amount of B_{12} than does maternal blood, even when maternal levels are depleted. Low maternal levels are associated with prematurity. The capacity of a woman to absorb B_{12} is increased during pregnancy and a large amount is transferred to the foetus. Vegetarian mothers have more chances of getting B_{12} deficiency. Serum levels drop during pregnancy and return to normal without supplementation after delivery. On the basis of the B_{12} content of foetuses, it has been estimated that foetal demands may be of the order of 0.3 *ug* per day.

Vitamin C

ICMR recommendations of vitamin C during pregnancy is 40 mg same as normal woman requirement. The foetal requirement is too small and sufficient safety margin is given for an adult women and extra allowance may not be necessary during pregnancy. In pregnancy vitamin C can fully cross the placental barrier. The vitamin C content of foetal blood is thrice as much as maternal blood. There is some evidence to show that the placenta can synthesize vitamin C. This may account for higher levels in foetal tissue. Low maternal intake of vitamin C is associated with premature rupture of foetal membranes and increased neonatal death rates.

A few studies have suggested an association between low plasma levels of vitamin C and preeclampsia.

Nutrient Status

- Nutrients given to fetus at the expense of mother-folacin, iron, vitamin C and B_{12}
- Nutrients for which mother and fetus compete- B_1, B_2, B_6 and D
- Nutrients for which mother has priority over fetus-vitamin A and I
- Nutrients stored in fetus-vitamin and iron
- Nutrients not stored in fetus- vitamin C,D and calcium

New Food Plan

For a pregnant woman whose diet has conformed to the "Basic Five Food" pattern, it is merely a matter of emphasising the more nutrient dense foods within each of the five food groups. Nutrient dense foods are those that give the most nutrients per calorie consumed. Most mothers are concerned enough about the health of their offspring and have a high motivation to eat right type of food. Pregnancy is perhaps the most effective time to attempt nutrition education.

Usually a daily diet containing 3 cups of milk or its equivalent, 2 servings of meat, fish, poultry eggs, or a source of complete protein, a dark-green or yellow vegetables and a generous serving of citrus fruits will provide a foundation for a nutritionally adequate diet. Between the 6th to 14th week of pregnancy 75 per cent women suffer from nausea which in turn affects their appetite. The consumption of small and frequent meals at regular intervals are helpful to many women. This pattern is also very helpful in the later part of pregnancy when discomfort is experienced after large meals due to over crowding by foetus in the abdominal cavity.

Eating a small meal just before hunger sensations usually become most severe, has been a useful method of controlling total intake. Intake must be maintained at steady levels so that the weight gain is not more than 400g/week, in the 2nd and 3rd trimesters of pregnancy. An erratic weight gain during pregnancy is associated with toxaemia and prematurity.

Impact of Nutritional Deficiency on Pregnancy

Nutrient	*Impact of deficiency on the*	
	Mother	*Infant*
Energy and Protein	• Abortion • Complications during delivery • Ketosis • May not gain enough weight to have normal lactation. • Oedema	• Premature infant • Low Birth weight Infant • Less brain cells

Contd...

Nutrient	*Impact of deficiency on the*	
	Mother	*Infant*
Linoleic Acid	—	• Foetal growth is affected
Calcium	• Muscular cramps Repeated pregnancy with poor diet can result in osteomalacia	• Calcification of bones and teeth is decreased
		• Underweight due to the decreased foetal bone growth.
	• During lactation breast milk may be deficient in calcium	
Iron	• Suffers from hypochromic microcytic anaemia.	• Born with less stores of iron and susceptible for anaemia.
	• Complications during delivery	
Sodium	• Increased risk of eclampsia	• Prematurity and low birth weight
Iodine	• Goitre	• Chance of getting goitre
	• Increased risk of miscarriage and still birth.	• Cretinism
Zinc	• Foetal mortality including central nervous system and teratogenecity.	• Reduced intra uterine
		• Foetal malformations growth rate
		• Low birth weight
		• Preterm baby.
Vitamin A	• Mortality	• Decreased levels in foetus so more susceptible for vitamin A deficiency.
Vitamin D	• Decreased calcium absorption.	• Calcium metabolism of foetus is affected.
Vitamin K	• Decreased prothrombin synthesis	• Increased risk of neonatal haemorrhage.

Contd...

Nutrient	*Impact of deficiency on the* Mother	*Impact of deficiency on the* Infant
	• Increased loss of blood during delivery.	
Thiamine, Riboflavin and Niacin.	• Energy deficiency symptoms.	
Folic acid	• Megaloblastic anaemia • Abrupto placenta	• Foetal malformation • Neural tube defects • Low Birth weight congenital abnormalities like hare lip, cleft palate, hydrocephalus.
Vitamin B_{12}	• Perminious anaemia	• Premature baby
Vitamin C.	• Premature rupture of foetal membranes.	• Increased neonatal death rate.

The selection of diet is also quite complicated because many women experience strong food dislikes and cravings. They often crave for foods they do not take ordinarily and develop strong distastes for foods they previously liked. In certain cases the aroma or sight (ads) to certain foods may evoke strong reactions. Mostly dislikes are oriented towards food that have no nutritional consequences. But if the dislike is for foods such as milk, which has good amounts of calcium then attention should be directed towards such an issue.

Plenty of water at least four to six glasses in addition to what is contained in the form of milk and other beverages should be taken daily throughout pregnancy. This will help keep the bowels regular. It has been found that infection of the tube connecting the kidney and bladder is less common among pregnant women who drink a lot of water. It is recommended that pregnant women limit their intake to 2 cups of caffeine containing beverages per day.

Faulty beliefs and wrong food habits need to be corrected during pregnancy.

Difficulties Involved

Nausea and Vomiting : Morning sickness of early pregnancy can be improved by small and frequent meals. Fairly dry and consisting chiefly of easily digested energy foods such as carbohydrates are more readily tolerated. Liquids may best be taken between meals instead of with food. If the condition develops to hyperemesis gravidarum, a severe prolonged persistent vomiting, peripheral parenteral nutrition and careful oral feeding is essential. Skim milk is better tolerated than whole milk. Fruits and vegetables can be given. Fatty rich foods, fried foods, excessive seasoning, coffee in large amounts and strongly flavoured vegetables may be restricted or eliminated if the nausea persists or if the patient complains of heartburn or gastric distress.

Constipation : The pressure of the enlarging uterus on the lower portion of the intestine, in addition to the hormonal muscle relaxant effect of placental hormones on the gastrointestinal tract and physical inactivity may make elimination difficult. Increased fluid intake and use of naturally laxative foods such as whole grains, dried fruits and other fruits, vegetables rich fibre, juices usually induce regularity, Laxatives should be avoided. Regular habits of exercise and sleep are essential for proper elimination.

Oedema and Leg Cramps : Mild, physiologic oedema is usually present in the extremities in the third trimester. The swelling of the lower extremities may be caused by the pressure of the enlarging uterus on the veins returning fluid from the legs. This normal oedema requires no sodium restriction or other dietary changes.

The common occurrence of cramps during pregnancy, manifested nocturnally by sudden contractions of the muscle, is thought to be related to a decline in serum calcium levels related to a calcium phosphorus imbalance. Prevention or relief of these leg cramps has been reported with reduction of milk (a high phosphorus, high calcium beverage) intake and supplementation with non-phosphate calcium salts. Magnesium is another mineral with the potential for relieving leg cramps.

Heart Burn : Heart burn is a common complaint during the latter part of pregnancy. In most cases, this is an effect of pressure of the enlarged uterus on the stomach which in combination with the relaxation of the oesophageal sphincter, results in occasional regurgitation of the stomach contents into the oesophagus. This can usually be relieved by limiting the amount of food consumed at one time and drinking fluids between meals. Sitting upright after meals for at least 3 hours before lying down may also help.

Beliefs, Avoidances, Cravings and Aversions : Food avoidances reflect mother's conscious choice not to consume certain foods during pregnancy e.g., heat producing foods like papaya and gingelly seeds.

Cravings and aversions are powerful urges toward or away from foods which women experience no unusual attitudes when not pregnant. The most commonly craved foods are sweets and dairy products. The most common aversions reported are to alcohol, coffee, other caffeinated drinks, meats and strongly spiced foods.

Consumption of non-food items like laundry starch, ice cubes or clay is called pica. It occurs more often during pregnancy than at any other time. The etiology of pica is poorly understood one theory suggests that the ingestion of non-food substances relieves nausea and vomiting. It has also been hypothesised that a deficiency for essential nutrient, such as calcium or iron, results in the eating of non-food substances that contain these nutrients. Much of this behaviour appears to be based on superstitions, customs and traditions that one often passes from mother to daughter.

Weight Gain during Pregnancy : All pregnancies should be started with BMI of 20-26 because maternal and foetal consequences occur at both extremes. Optimal weight gain is about 11 to 13 kg. About 900 to 1800 g is an average gain during the first trimester. Thereafter 450 g/week during the remainder of the pregnancy is usual. Sharp sudden increase in weight after the 20th week of pregnancy, which may indicate excessive, abnormal water retention should be watched. Weight reduction should never be undertaken during pregnancy. Excessive weight gain places an extra strain on the organs and increases the incidence to toxaemia. It is not correct for the mother to think that low gain in weight results in smaller baby which is easy to deliver.

Tables below give the components of weight gain during pregnancy and recommended weight gain based on body mass index.

Components of Weight Gain during Pregnancy - 28-40 Weeks

Component	*Weight g*
Foetus	3000
Placenta and amniotic acid	1500
Maternal tissues and blood	7000
Total	11500

Recommended Weight Gains for Pregnant Women based on Body Mass Index

Weight category	*Total weight*
Based on BMI	***gain (kg)***
Under weight (BMI < 19.8)	12.5- 18
Normal weight (19.8 - 26)	11.5 - 16
Overweight BMI > 26 - 29	7-11.5
Obese > 29	6.0

Research shows that continuing a regular exercise regimen throughout pregnancy is helpful in improved fitness, prevention of gestational diabetes, facilitation of labour and reduced stress.

Anaemia : Physiological changes in the blood occur progressively during normal pregnancy. Haemoglobin mass increases, red blood cell volume increases, plasma volume rises and haemoglobin concentration drops from 13.4 to 11.6 g per 100 ml. Severe anaemia in pregnant women increases maternal morbidity and mortality and involves a higher risk of the foetus. A pregnant woman is labelled anaemic if from the 28th week onwards the haemoglobin is less than 10 g per 100 ml of blood.

A significant fall in birth weight due to increase in prematurity rate and intrauterine growth retardation has been reported to occur when maternal haemoglobin level falls below 8g/dl. Anaemic pregnant women are prone to urinary infections. The effect of anaemia and urinary tract infection in pregnancy could also be the cause of low birth weight infant.

The predominantly cereal diet in the tropics should be able to provide 40 mg iron per day. Treatment of highly deficient states requires daily therapeutic doses of 120 to 200 mg. This oral therapy may be continued for 3-6 months after anaemia has been corrected in order to replenish the depleted stores. Administration orally of 60 mg elemental iron and 500 *ug* of folk acid per day in the last trimester of pregnancy prevents anaemia.

The demand for folate is increased because of increased cellular proliferation. The low folate levels are due to deficient intake. Folates are easily destroyed by cooking, hence fresh vegetables should be included in the diet of pregnant woman. Megaloblastic anaemia results in intensified nausea, vomiting and anorexia. Five mg of folic acid supplement ensures an adequate supply for prophylactic purposes.

Anaemia due to B_{12} deficiency in pregnancy is uncommon. A single injection of 40 mcg of B_{12} is enough to produce a maximum response in 10 days in B_{12} deficient mothers.

Pregnancy Induced Hypertension (toxaemia) : Studies conducted at National Institute of Nutrition (1992-93) indicate that severe pregnancy induced hypertension (eclampsia) are associated with higher incidence of vitamin A and protein deficiencies resulting in poor pregnancy outcome.

It is common among women subsisting on inadequate diets with little or no prenatal care. The symptoms of PIH include hypertension, abnormal and excessive oedema, albuminuria, convulsions or coma. Optimal nutrition is a fundamental aspect of therapy. Emphasis is given to adequate dietary protein. Correction of plasma protein deficits stimulates normal operation of the capillary fluid shift mechanism and circulation of fluid tissue with subsequent correction of the hypovolaemia (abnormal reduction in volume of circulatory plasma). In addition, adequate salt and sources of vitamins and minerals are needed for correction and maintenance of metabolic balance.

Hypertension : This can cause considerable maternal and foetal consequences. Nutritional therapy will centre on (1) prevention of weight extremes, underweight or obesity (2) correction of any dietary deficiencies and maintenance of optimal nutritional status during pregnancy and (3) management of any related preexisting disease such as diabetes mellitus. Sodium intake may be moderate but should not be unduly restricted.

Diabetes Mellitus : During pregnancy glycosuria is not uncommon, because of the increased circulating blood volume and its load of metabolites. Most of these women revert to normal glucose tolerance after delivery.

Dietary Guidelines

- Small and frequent feedings should be taken. Avoid fasting or missing any meal.
- More fibre should be included in the diet to prevent constipation which is a common problem during pregnancy. 5-6 Servings of fruits and vegetables should be included in the daily diet.
- Diet should be rich in calcium to prevent osteomalacia. Calcium supplements may also be taken.
- Iron rich foods should be taken to prevent anaemia and to build up iron stores in the foetal body. Iron supplements may be taken.
- Diet should contain optimum amount of sodium. In case of oedema or hypertension, sodium is restricted.
- Inclusion of green leafy vegetables ensures minerals like calcium and iron.
- Plenty of water should be taken to keep the bowels regular.
- Fatty rich foods, fried foods, excessive seasoning, strongly flavoured vegetables may be restricted in case of nausea and gastric distress.
- Fluids should be taken between meals rather than along with the meals.
- Adequate amount of calories should be taken so that enough fat is deposited during pregnancy which is required for lactation.

WHO and UNICEF have repeatedly emphasised that too early pregnancies (teenager), too late (35 and over), too close (less than two years) and too many (four and over) are not safe or conducive to the health of either the mother or her infant.

Some Suggested Recipes during Pregnancy

Recipes	*Reason*
Dairy products like milk, curd, khoya, yogurt and cheese, paneer	To meet the requirements of protein, calcium and vitamin D and to prevent muscle cramps
Banana, green leafy vegetables, whole grain cereals	Natural laxatives and prevent constipation.
Fruit salad	Appetising and provide many nutrients and also fibre.
Omlette, boiled egg, scrambled egg, liver curry	Good quality protein and iron
Rice flakes upma, puffed rice ball	Good source of iron and easy to digest
Green gram, dal, pakoda, bread pudding, carrot halwa	Nutrient dense foods to be given to meet increased requirements.
Pickles, rasam, sour foods	These foods may give relief from nausea.

13

Treatment by Diet

Dietics is a science that deals with the adequacy of diets during normal life cycle and modifications required during diseased conditions. Menu planning is the process of planning and scheduling intake of meals for a general or specific individual requirements. The following terms and concepts are widely used and a clear understanding of these terms makes menu planning efficient.

The Fundamentals

Health is defined by the World Health Organisation of the United Nations as the "State of complete physical, mental and social well being and not merely the absence of disease and infirmity."

The essential requisites (or dimensions) of "health" would include the following:

* Achievement of optimal growth and development, reflecting the full expression of one's genetic potential.
* Maintenance of the structural integrity and functional efficiency of body tissues necessary for an active and productive life.

* Mental well-being.
* Ability to withstand the inevitable process of ageing with minimal disability and functional impairment, and
* Ability to combat disease, such as

a. resisting infections (immunocompetence)

b. preventing the onset (and retarding the progress) of degenerative diseases and cancer and

c. resisting the effect of environmental toxins and pollutants.

Nutrient requirement can be defined as the minimum amount of the absorbed nutrient that is necessary for maintaining the normal physiological functions of the body.

Recommended Dietary Allowances (RDA) is defined as the nutrient present in the diet which satisfies the daily requirement of nearly all individuals in a population. These imply addition of safety factor amount to the estimated requirement to cover the variation among individuals, losses during cooking and the lack of precision inherent in the estimated requirement.

Recommended Dietary Allowances = Requirements + Safety factor.

Recommended Dietary Allowances of an individual depends on many factors like age, sex, physical work and physiological stress.

* *Age:* An adult requires more total calories than a child due to larger size of the body and increase in activity. A growing child requires more calories and protein per kilogram of body weight than an adult.
* *Sex:* Females require less calories than males as BMR is lower and size of the body is smaller.
* *Physical Work:* Sedentary workers require less calories and B-vitamins than hard working persons.
* *Physiological Stress:* During pregnancy and lactation period the requirement of nutrients are increased.

Adequate intake (AI) is a nutrient recommendation based on observed or experimentally determined approximation of nutrient intake by a group of healthy people when sufficient scientific evidence is not available to calculate an RDA.

Balanced diet is one which contains different types of foods in such quantities and proportions so that the need for calories, proteins, minerals, vitamins and other nutrients is adequately met and a small provision is made for extra nutrients to withstand short duration of leanness.

In addition a balanced diet should provide bio-active phyto-chemicals such as dietary fibre, antioxidants and nutraceuticals which have positive health benefits.

A balanced diet should provide around 60-70% of total calories from carbohydrate, 10-12% from protein and 20-25% of total calories from fat.

Herbal Elements

Dietary fibre is defined as that portion of food derived from plant cells, which is resistant to hydrolysis/digestion and consists of hemicellulose, cellulose, lignins, oligosaccharides, pectins, gums and waxes.

Fibre is helpful in preventing constipation, coronary heart diseases, diabetes mellitus, obesity and colonic cancer.

Whole grain cereals like ragi, wheat and whole pulses like blackgram are good sources of dietary fibre. Green leafy vegetables, fruits and skins and seeds also contribute to the fibre content of the diet.

Diet Plan

Antioxidants : The normal fụnctioning of cells is dependent on a proper balance of pro-oxidant and antioxidants. The former promote the release of oxygen to provide the energy needed for cell functioning. Antioxidants help to neutralise and counteract the deleterious free radicals but the natural mechanisms may prove to be inadequate. Especially in poor environments, in addition to free radicals, generated as part of the natural metabolic process, the body also has to deal with free radical species derived from such environmental contaminants as smoke, carcinogenic chemicals derived from food additives and industrial effluent and radiation.

Free radicals could promote lipid peroxidation of membrane lipids impairing cell function, they could damage cellular proteins and DNA; they could cause peroxidation of circulating lipoprotein lipids thus converting them into the more deleterious form. Cumulative tissue injury thus caused by free radicals is now known to underlie the pathogenesis of such diverse conditions as cancer, atherosclerosis and heart diseases, radiation damage and accelerated ageing.

Enzyme antioxidants are superoxide dismutase, (Mn-containing superoxide dismutase, Cu-zn containing superoxide dismutase), glutathione peroxidase (selenium dependent), glutathione -S-transferase, glutathione reductase and catalase.

Coenzyme antioxidants are vitamin A, C, and E, and ubiquinol (reduced form of coenzyme Q).

Some nutrients such as carotenoids, ascorbic acid and tocopherols possess antioxidant properties thus playing a dual role. Prominent common foods possessing such antioxidant activity are green leafy vegetables, fruits like amla and guava, palm oil and sunflower oil and spices like turmeric and cloves.

Diet Therapy

Nutraceuticals : The word combines "nutrition" and "pharmaceuticals" to mean that food extracts can be used as preventive drugs or food supplements.

The major phyto-nutrients identified to have nutraceutical properties include terpenes, phytosterol, phenols and theols.

Terpenes represent the largest class of phyto-nutrients. They are found in green foods, soya products and grains. Carotenoids and limonoids are the two major terpene sub-classes. Carrots, tomatoes, parsley, orange and spinach are rich sources of carotenoids. They act as vitamin A precursor and have preventive action against many eye diseases. They can also prevent the oxidation of vitamin A and E. Limonoids act as antioxidants protecting lung tissues from free oxygen. Citrus peel can act as nutraceuticals supplying limonoids.

Phytosterols form another major class of phyto-nutrients, which are present in all plants. However, the rich sources having nutraceutical functions include yellow vegetables, seeds of pumpkins and yams. This phyto chemical competes with dietary cholesterol for uptake in the intestine thereby blocking cholesterol absorption into the body. It facilitates the excretion of cholesterol from the body. It can also prevent the development of tumour in breast and prostate glands.

Flavonoides are phyto-chemicals that enhance the effectiveness of vitamin C. They can also act against allergies, ulcers, tumours and platelet aggregation. They are effective in controlling high blood pressure and can reduce the risk of oestrogen induced cancer.

Anthocyanidins or flavonals have significant role in collagen protein synthesis. They are important in sports medicine also. Athletes who exercise excessively produce free radicals that are tackled by anthocyanidins.

Isoflavones can prevent tumour growth. Beans and other legumes are rich sources with nutraceutical properties. Important isoflavones, genestein and daidzin found in soyabeans have nutraceutical properties against tumour growth. People who consume soya food rarely experience breast, uterus and prostate cancer.

Theols are a major sulphur containing class of phyto-nutrients. The food sources having theolic nutraceutical properties include garlic, onions, mustard and other cruciferous vegetables like cabbage and turnip. Important sub-classes under theols are glucosinolates, allelic sulphides, indoles, isoprenoids and tocopherols. Cruciferous vegetables form rich sources of glucosinolates. They activate liver detoxification enzymes and can reduce the incidence of tumor.

Allelic sulphides are potent antimutagenic and anti-carcinogenic agents. They protect against tumours and give cardiovascular protection. They can block the activity of toxins produced by bacteria and viruses, thereby building immunity against diseases.

Isoprenoids are active against free radicals in the body. Thus they reduce oxidative damage of tissues. Tocopherols found in grains and palm oil inhibit breast cancer.

Probiotics and Prebiotics : Probiotics are live microbial food or feed supplements that benefit human and animal health by improving the microbial balance in the intestine.

Prebiotics promote the growth of probiotics in the form of specific substrates.

Products containing both probiotics and prebiotics are being commercially produced.

Collective Steps

The five food group plan permits an individual to plan a menu to achieve nutrient intakes as specified by RDA. The five food groups suggested by ICMR are given in Table below.

The Five Food Groups and their Major Nutrients

Food Group	*Main Nutrients*
1. Cereal grains and products: Wheat, Ragi, Bajra, Maize, Jowar, Barley, Rice flakes, wheat flour	Energy, Protein, Invisible fat, Vitamin-B1 Rice, Vitamin-B_2 Folic acid, Iron, Fibre.
2. Pulses and Legumes: Bengalgram, Blackgram, Greengram, Cowpea, Peas, Rajmah, Soyabean, Beans.	Energy, Protein, Invisible fat, Vitamin-B_1, Vitamin-B_2 Folic acid, Calcium, Iron, Fibre. Redgram, Lentil (whole as well as dals),
3. Milk and Meat Products: Milk, Curd, Skimmed Milk, Cheese, Chicken, Liver, Fish, Egg, Meat	Protein, Fat, Vitamin-B_2, Calcium
4. Fruits and Vegetables:	Carotenoids, Vitamin-C, Fibre,
Fruits: Mango, Guava, Tomato, Papaya, Orange, Sweet lime, Water melon.	Invisible fat, Vitamin-B_2, Folic acid, Iron.
Vegetables: (green leafy) Amaranth, Spinach, Gogu, Drumstick leaves, Coriander leaves, Fenugreek leaves.	Carotenoids Vitamin-B_2, Folic Acid, Calcium, Iron, Fibre.
Other Vegetables: Carrots, Brinjal, Ladies finger, Beans Capsicum, Onion, Drumstick, Cauliflower.	Carotenoids, Folic acid, Calcium, Fibre
5. Fats and Sugar:	Energy, Fat, Essential Fatty acids.
Fats: Butter, Ghee, Hydrogenated fat,	
Cooking oils like groundnut, Mustard,	
Coconut Sugar: Jaggery and sugar	Energy

The five food group system can be used by health professionals for the following purposes:

1. *Tool for Nutritional Assessment and Screenings:* A brief dietary history system can disclose inadequacies of nutrient from any of the five groups. The information can be the first clue for the possibility of the subject may be at the risk of developing nutritional deficiency.
2. *Tool for Nutritional Counselling:* The dietary history based on the five food group system allows a health team to counsel or teach a patient about nutrition.
3. *Explaining Therapeutic Diets to the Patient:* Therapeutic diets are scientifically based on nutrient composition and groups which can be used in menu planning.
4. *Food Labelling and Surveillance System:* Food groups can be used for food labelling and for nutrition surveillance system.

The Principles

a. *Meeting Nutritional Requirement: A* good menu is one which will not only provide adequate calories, fat and proteins but also minerals, vitamins essential for the physical well being of each member of a family. In a balanced diet the ratio of energy distribution from carbohydrate, protein and fat would be 7:1:2. The diet should contain 'Basic five food groups'.
b. *Meal Pattern must Fulfill Family Needs:* A family meal should cater to the needs of the different members. A growing adolescent boy may need rich food to satisfy his appetite, whereas a young child may require soft and bland diet. Pregnant women require more greens in the diet. A heavy worker requires more calories and B vitamins than other members of the family. Meal pattern varies with age, occupation and life-style of the family members.
c. *Meal Planning should save time and Energy:* Planning of meals should be done in such a way, that the recipes should be simple and nutritious. By using Basic Five Food Groups, time can be saved.
d. *Economic Consideration:* Any meals that are planned, if do not satisfy the budget of the family, it cannot be put into practice. The cost of meals can be reduced by using seasonal

foods, by bulk purchasing and substituting greens for fruits.

e. *Meal Plan should give Maximum Nutrients:* Losses of nutrients during processing, cooking should be minimised. Sprouted grams, malted cereals, fermented foods enhance the nutritive value. Good quality protein should be distributed in all meals. Pressure cooker can be used to conserve the nutrients.

f. *Consideration for Individual Likes and Dislikes:* The meal planned should not only meet RDA but also individual preferences, particularly vegetarian or non-vegetarian preferences. If a person does not like particular greens, it can be tried in a different form or substituted by some other equally nourishing food. Food habits and dietary pattern should also be considered. Religion, traditions and customs of the individual should be considered in planning the menu.

g. *Planned Meals should Provide Variety:* If the meals are monotonous it is not consumed. Variety can be introduced in colour, texture and taste, by using different kinds of foods and cooking methods. Variety also helps in meeting the nutritional requirement.

h. *Meals should give Satiety:* Each meal should have some amount of fat, protein and fibre to get satiety. Meals should be planned in such a way that interval between the meals is also considered.

i. *Availability of Foods:* Menus should include locally available foods. The wide variation in dietary patterns throughout the world depends largely upon the available food supply.

Points to be Considered : For planning the menu the following points should be considered:

* Variety of foods should be used in the menu. No single food has all the nutrients.
* Caloric allowance can be 50±. For all other nutrients minimum RDA must be met.
* Energy derived from cereals should be not more than 75 per cent.

* Whole grain cereals, parboiled grains or malted grains give higher nutritive value.
* It is better to include two cereals in one meal like rice and wheat or millets and rice.
* Flour should not be sieved for Chapati as it reduces bran content.
* To improve the cereal and pulse protein quality minimum ratio of cereal protein to pulse protein should be 4 :1. In terms of the grains it will be 8 parts of cereals and one part of pulses.
* Two to 3 servings of pulses should be taken every day.
* Green leafy vegetables can be taken more than one serving, if fruit is not included in the diet.
* Foods rich in fibre should be included in the diet.
* It is better to serve the fruit raw without much cooking or taking juice out of it. Every diet should contain atleast one medium size fruit.
* There should be a minimum milk of 100 ml/day. One to two glasses of milk or curd should be included in a balanced diet.
* Energy derived from fats or oils is 15-20 per cent of total calories and 5 per cent from sugar and jaggery.
* One egg weighs around 40 g. This can be served along with cereal or pulses to improve the quality of protein. Instead, one serving of poultry/fish can also be included in the diet.
* Inclusion of salads or raita not only helps in meeting the vitamin requirements but the meals would be attractive and have high satiety value due to the fibre content.
* Fried foods cannot be planned if oil allowance is less or in low calorie diets.
* One-third of nutritional requirement—at least calories and protein should be met by lunch or dinner.
* If possible, meals should be planned at a time for several days.

* Usually the number of meals would be four and for very young children and patients, number of meals can be more.
* Ideally each meal should consist of all the five food groups.
* For quick calculations food exchange list can be used.
* Balanced diet should meet antioxidant requirement.
* Processed foods contain a variety of food additives. They may not be nutritionally balanced unless fortified.
* Five servings of fruits and vegetables should be included in a day's diet.

Steps Involved : There are three steps involved in planning a menu

Step I—Recommended Dietary Allowances : To calculate balanced diet, as a first step there is a need to know Recommended Dietary Allowances for different age groups prescribed by Nutrition Expert Committee of ICMR. Table below shows Recommended Dietary Allowances for Indians (1989).

Step II—Food List : Food list can be prepared either by using ICMR Tables or Exchange lists.

Using ICMR Tables : As a second step while planning the daily diet the foods are chosen from all five food groups. To make menu planning more convenient ICMR has suggested the portion size and balanced diets for adults and for different age groups.

The balanced diets for adults and different age groups are given as multiples of these portion sizes.

Using Exchange Lists : The diet can also be prescribed in terms of exchange lists. Food exchange lists are groups of measured foods of the same calorific value and similar protein, fat and carbohydrate. In the same group one can be substituted for the other. All foods of exchange lists make a specific contribution to a good diet. None of the exchange groups can itself supply all the nutrients needed for a well balanced diet. Each exchange provides 100 kcals.

There is no fat exchange as the calorie value of the recipes include fat that is used. If additional fat or sugar is used, calorie value can be calculated by multiplying with 9 or 4 per gram respectively.

Recommended dietary allowances for Indians—1989

Group	Particulars	Body wt	Net energy	Protein	Fat	Calcium	Iron	Vitamin A: Retinol	Vitamin A: β-carotene	Thiamine	Riboflavin	Nicotinic acid	Pyridoxin	Ascorbic acid	Folic acid	Vit. B_{12}
		kg	Kcal/d	g/d	g/d	mg/d	mg/d	μg/d	μg/d	mg/d	mg/d	mg/d	mg/d	mg/d	μg/d	μg/d
Man	Sedentary work		2425							1.2	1.4	16				
	Moderate work	60	2875	60	20	400	28	600	2400	1.4	1.6	18	2.0	40	100	1
	Heavy work		3800							1.6	1.9	21				
Women	Sedentary work		1875							0.9	1.1	12				
	Moderate work	50	2225	50	20	400	30	600	2400	1.1	1.3	14	2.0	40	100	1
	Heavy work		2925							1.2	1.5	16				
	Pregnant woman		+300	+15	30	1000	38	600	2400	+0.2	+0.2	+2	2.5	40	400	1
	Lactation															
	0-6 months	50	+550	+25						+0.3	+0.3	+4				
	6-12 months		+400	+18	45	1000	30	950	3800	+0.2	+0.2	+3	2.5	80	150	1.5
Infants	0-6 months	5.4	108/kg	2.05/kg		500				55μg/kg	65μg/kg	710μg/kg	0.1	25	25	0.2
	6-12 months	8.6	98/kg	1.65/kg				350	1400	50μg/kg	60μg/kg	650μg/kg	0.4			
Children	1-3 years	12.2	1240	22			12	400		0.6	0.7	8	0.9		30	
	4-6 years	19.0	1690	30	25	400	18	400	1600	0.9	1.0	11		40	40	0.2-1.0
	7-9 years	26.9	1950	41			26	600	2400	1.0	1.2	13	1.6		60	
Boys	10-12 years	35.4	2190	54			34			1.1	1.3	15				
Girls	10-12 years	31.5	1970	57	22	600	19	600	2400	1.0	1.2	13	1.6	40	70	0.2-1.0
Boys	13-15 years	47.8	2450	70			41			1.2	1.5	16				
Girls	13-15 years	46.7	2060	65	22	600	28	600	2400	1.0	1.2	14	2.0	40	100	0.2-1.0
Boys	16-18 years	57.1	2640	78			50			1.3	1.6	17				
Girls	16-18 years	49.9	2060	63	22	500	30	600	2400	1.0	1.2	14	2.0	40	100	0.2-1.0

Source: Gopalan C., B.V. Rama Sastri and S.C. Balasubramanian 1991, Nutritive Value of Indian Foods, National Institute of Nutrition, ICMR, Hyderabad 500 007, India.

Portion size for Menu Plan

Food groups	Portion g	Energy kcal	Protein g	Carbohydrate g	Fat g
Cereals and Millets	30	100	3.0	20	0.8
Pulses	30	100	6.0	15	0.7
Egg	50	85	7.0	—	7.0
Meat, Chicken or fish	50	100	9	—	7.0
Milk	100	70	3.0	5	3.0
Roots and Tubers	100	80	1.3	19	—
Green leafy vegetables	100	45	3.6	-	0.4
Other vegetables	100	30	1.7	-	0.2
Fruits	100	40	—	10	—
Sugar	5	20	—	5	—
Fats & Oils	5	45	—	—	5

Balanced Diet for Adults—sedentary/moderate/heavy Activity (number of portions)

Food Groups	Portion	Type of work					
	g	Sedentary		Moderate		Heavy	
		Man	Woman	Man	Woman	Man	Woman
Cereals and millets	30	14	10	16	12	23	16
Pulses	30	2	2	3	2.5	3	3
Milk	100 ml	3	3	3	3	3	3
Roots & tubers	100	2	1	2	1	2	2
Green leafy vegetables	100	1	1	1	1	1	1
Other vegetables	100	1	1	1	1	1	1
Fruits	100	1	1	1	1	1	1
Sugar	5	5	4	8	5	11	9
Fats and Oils (visible)	5	4	4	7	6	11	8

For non-vegetarians substitute one pulse portion with one portion of egg/meat/chicken/ fish.

Recipes from exchange lists are selected from all groups and energy and protein value are calculated in accordance with the RDA. If specific number of exchange lists are chosen from each group and energy and protein RDA are met, most of the time all the other nutrients are also met.

Step III: Making the Menu : The foods that are listed in step II are converted into the actual recipes and distributed in different meals like breakfast, lunch, evening tea and dinner. Recipes in exchange lists are distributed in different meals.

Balanced diet for infants, children and adolescents (number of portions)

Food Groups	*Portion g*	*Infants 6-12 months*	*Years*						
			1-3	*4-6*	*7-9*	*10-12*		*13-18*	
						Girls	*Boys*	*Girls*	*Boys*
Cereals and millets	30	1.5	4	7	9	9	11	10	14
Pulses	30	0.5	1	1.5	2	2	2	2	2
Milk (ml)	100	5*	5	5	5	5	5	5	5
Roots & tubers	100	0.5	0.5	1	1	1	1	1	2
Green leafy vegetables	100	0.25	0.5	0.5	1	1	1	1	1
Other vegetables	100	0.25	0.5	0.5	1	1	1	1	1
Fruits	100	1	1	1	1	1	1	1	1
Sugar	5	5	5	6	6	6	7	6	7
Fats/Oils (Visible)	5	2	4	5	5	5	5	5	5

*Quantity indicates top milk. For breast-fed infants, 200 ml top milk is required.

One portion of pulse may be exchanged with one portion (50 g) of egg/meat/chicken/fish.

For infants introduce egg/meat/chicken/fish around 9 months. Specific recommendations as compared to a sedentary woman:

Children

1-6 years	:	½ to 3/4 the amount of cereals, pulses and vegetables and extra cup of milk.
7-12 years	:	Extra cup of milk
Adolescent girls	:	Extra cup of milk
Adolescent boys	:	Diet of sedentary man with extra cup of milk.

100 kcal. exchange list

capacity of one standard katori is 130 ml.

Cereal exchange - 1.5 - 3.5 g protein

Idli (big)	1
(medium)	1½
Dosa (small)	1
(big)	½
Phulka	2
Chapati	1
Puri	1½
Rava Idli	1
Veg. Sandwich	¾
Bread Toast (medium)	1½
Plain rice	¾ K
Upma	1½ K
Veg. Noodles	1 K
Naan	⅔
Cheese Sandwich	⅓
Ragi puttu	¾ K
Ragi adai	¾
Pulao	½ K
Bise bela bath	½ K

Tamarind rice	½ K
Curd rice	½ K
Pulse Exchange 3-5 g protein	
Sambar	1½ K
Rasam	2½ K
Thickdal	½ K
Thin dal	1 K
Channa masala	½ K
Dry peas sundal	¾ K
Roasted Bengal gram chutney (without coconut)	½ K
Sprouted moong salad	1 heaped katori
Pesarattu	¾
Baked Masala Vada (with negligible amount of fat)	2 nos
Adai	1
Vada	1
Bajji	2
Milk exchange - 4.5 g protein	
Milk	150 ml - 1 tea cup
Curd	150 ml - 1 full katori
Cheese	1 ⅓ cube 30g
Paneer	40 g
Butter milk	1 glass - (350 ml)
Milk kheer	½ K
Meat exchange 5 g of protein	
Egg omelette	1
Scrambled egg	One egg
Fish Kolambu	⅔ K

Fish fry	1 small piece
Boiled egg with gravy	⅓ to ½ serving
Meat curry	1 serving
Vegetable A exchange	
Curry without coconut and gravy (with simple seasoning)	1 heaped Katori
Plain tomato soup	2 K (1 soup bowl)
Soup with white sauce	1 K (½ soup bowl)
Mint chutney	7½ tsp.
Mixed vegetable chowder	¾ C
Vegetable B exchange	
Roots and tubers curry	½ K
Cutlet	½ K
Fruit exchange	
Apple	1 medium
Banana	1
Orange	2½
Sapota	2 (small)
Fruit salad (no sugar or dressing)	¾ K
Guava	1 (Big)

The Pyramid : The food guide pyramid is an educational tool that shows the dietary guidelines in the easily understood graphic format. It was originally prepared by the Human Nutrition Information Service and published in 1992 by the U.S. Department of Agriculture. It is meant for use by the general healthy population as a guide for the amounts and types of foods to be included in the daily diet. The pyramid was designed to help teach the concepts of variety, moderation and the inclusion of food types in appropriate proportion in the total diet. The food guide pyramid can be modified for different age groups.

The numbers in the figure indicates the exchanges required of the group by an adult man doing sedentary work.

Herbal Eatables

Vegetarian Diets : Vegetarian diets consist of foods of plant origin. The two classic variants are lacto-ovo-vegetarian and strict vegetarian or vegan. There are a number of dietary, religious and moral considerations which may lead individuals to limit or modify the vegetarian diet. In India most of the population are vegetarians due to economic reasons. Vegetarians should include variety of plant foods like grains, legumes, ruts and seeds to meet the nutritional requirement. Those whose nutrient needs are especially high due to growth, pregnancy, lactation, or recovery from illness can generally meet their nutrient requirements on well planned vegetarian diet containing dairy products.

Foods like greens and gingelly seeds are good calcium but all may not be available due to the presence of oxalates and phybates. Lacto vegetarians can get plenty of calcium from milk and milk products. Good plant food sources of iron include dried beans, dark green vegetables, dried fruits and iron fortified cereals. To enhance absorption of iron a good source of ascorbic acid with meals is indicated. Classifications of vegetarian diet and nutritional adequacy is given in Table below

Classification of Vegetarianism

Classification	*Foods Included*	*Foods Excluded*	*Limiting Nutrients*
Semi-vegetarian	Fruits, grains, legumes, nuts, vegetables, seeds, milk, milk products, eggs, chicken, fish	All other animal meat	
Pesco-vegetarian	Fruits, grains, legumes, nuts, seeds, vegetables, milk, milk products, eggs and fish	Animal meat	
Lacto-ovo-vegetarian	Fruits, grains, legumes, nuts, seeds, vegetables, milk, milk products	Animal meat and eggs	Iron

Contd...

Classification	*Foods Included*	*Foods Excluded*	*Limiting Nutrients*
Lacto-vegetarian	Fruits, grains, legumes, nuts, seeds, vegetables, milk, milk products	Animal meat and eggs	Iron
Ovo-vegetarian	Fruits, grains, legumes, nuts, seeds, vegetables, and eggs	Animal meat, milk, and products	Vitamin D, calcium, riboflavin, iron
Vegan	Fruits, grains, legumes, nuts, seeds, vegetables	All animal products	High quality protein, sufficient calories, vitamin D, B-12, and riboflavin, iron and calcium

Vitamin B_{12} is found in animal foods. Meeting the requirement of vitamin B_{12} is not a concern for most vegetarians who consume dairy products or eggs. It is a concern for vegans and supplement of vitamin B_{12} to their diets is necessary.

For vegans, special care must be taken to ensure adequacy of vitamin D, iron and vitamin B_{12} and if necessary supplementation may be necessary.

Vegetarian diet is a good source of fibre. Vegetarians usually have faster gastrointestinal transit time, bulkier stools and low serum cholesterol levels. In general, coronary heart disease, high blood pressure, type II diabetes, obesity and some forms of cancer tend to develop less often in vegetarians than in non-vegetarians. Lacto vegetarian diet is a low risk diet for colon cancer, oesophageal cancer.

Bibliography

Ansell, G.B. : *Functions of Phospholipids*, Elsevier, New York, 1973.

Ashworth, G. : *Recreation and Hotel Management*, Bell and Hyman, London, 1984.

Austin, A. and A. Ram : *Studies on Chapati-Making Quality of Wheat*, Indian Council of Agricultural Research, New Delhi, 1971.

Barrow, G.M. : *Physical Chemistry for Life Science*, McGraw-Hill Book Company, New York, 1992.

Bernecker, Paul : *Methods and Hotel Industry*, Austrian National Tourist Office, Vienna, 1961.

Bharathi, V.V. : *Anxiety Behaviour in Children*, Discovery Publishing House, New Delhi, 1992.

Bhatia, K. H. :*Hotel Management and Marketing*, Sterling, New Delhi, 1997.

Boniface, B and Cooper, C. : *The Geography of Travel and Tourism*, Heinemann, London, 1987.

Brunner, E. : *Holiday Making and the Holiday Trades*, Oxford University Press, London, 1945.

Burkart, A.J. : *The Management of Tourism*, Heinemann, London, 1975.

Cambell, A.M., M.P. Penfield, and R.M. Griswold : *Experimental Study of Foods*, Houghton, 1990.

Charalambons, G., and G. Inglett : *The Quality of Foods and Beverages: Chemistry and Technology*, Academic Press, New York, 1981.

Cherry, J.P. : *Protein Functionality in Foods*, American Chemical Society, Washington D.C., 1981.

Clare, Gunn : *Hotel Management Planning*, Taylor and Francis, New York, 1988.

Clayne, R. Jensen : *Leisure and Recreation : Introduction to Hotel Management*, Lea and Febiger, Philadelphia, 1977.

Colley, G. : *International Hotel Management Today*, Lloyds Bank Review, London, 1967.

Crampon, L.T. : *An Analysis of Tourist Markets*, University of Colorado Press, Colorado, 1963.

Dale, E. : *Management Theory and Practice*, McGraw-Hill, New York, 1973.

Davidson, R. : *Hotel Industry in Europe*, Pitman, London, 1992.

Davis, H.D. : *Potentials for Tourism of Developing Countries*, Finance and Development, London, 1968.

Dharamraj, E. : *Food and Hotel Legislations and Policies*, New Age Publishers, New Delhi, 1998.

Douglas, Pearce : *Tourism Today : A Geographical Analysis*, Longman, New York, 1987.

Dumazedier, J. : *Towards a Society of Leisure*, Free Press, New York, 1967.

Ed Gell, D. L. : *International Hotel Industry Policy*, Van Nostrand Reinhold, New York, 1990.

Edwards, Francis, G. : *How to Focus ? Your Marketing Efforts*, Louis A. Allen Associates, London, 1976.

Feiffer, M. : *Giving Places*, MacMillan, London, 1985.

Forrest, J.C., E.D. Aberle, H.B. Hedrick, M.D. Judge and R.A Merkel : *Principles of Meat Science*, W.H. Freeman and Co., San Francisco, 1975.

Frank, R.E. : *Market Segmentation*, Prentice-Hall, New Jersey, 1972.

Gill, Pushpinder S. : *Tourism and Hotel Management*, Anmol Publications, New Delhi, 1996.

Gunn, C. : *Tourism Planning*, Taylor and Francis, New York, 1988.

Gyorgy, P. and W.N. Pearson : *The Vitamin*, Academic Press, New York, 1967.

Hascherneyer, R. and A.H. Haschemeyer : *Proteins : A Guide to Study of Physical and Chemical Methods*, John Wiley & Sons, New York, 1973.

Hiller, Herbet L. : *The Development of Tourism in the Caribbean Region*, Air Travel and Tourism, New York, 1972.

Holloway, J. C. : *Marketing or Tourism*, Longman, Harlow, 1995.

Hudson, E. : *Vertical Integration in Travel and Leisure Industry*, Institute of Air Transport, Paris, 1972.

Ian M. Matley : *The Geography of International Tourism*, Association of American Geographers, Washington, 1976.

Jefferson, A. : *Marketing Tourism*, Longman, Harlow, 1988.

John, Lea : *Hotel Industry Development in the Third World*, Routledge, New York, 1988.

Kacharoo, P. : *Pulse Crops of India*, ICAR, New Delhi, 1970.

Katler, P. : *Introduction to Marketing Management, Analysis, Planning and Control*, Prentice-Hall, London, 1975.

Kotler, P. : *Theory of Cookery*, Prentice-Hall, London, 1975.

Krippendorf, J. : *The Holiday Makers, Understanding the Impact of Leisure and Travel*, Heinemann, Oxford, 1987.

Kusuma, D.L. : *Profile of Nutrition of Rural Adolescent Girls*, Discovery Publishing House, New Delhi, 2001.

Lal, H. : *Total Quality Management : A practical Approach*, New Age Publishers, New Delhi, 2000.

Lansing, J.B. Blood, D.M. : *The Changing Travel Market*, University of Michigan, Michigan, 1964.

Lawson, Malcom : *Teaching Hotel Management Education and Training in Western Europe: A Comparative Study*, Tourism International Press, London, 1975.

Lickorish, L. J. : *Hotel Industry and International Balance of Payments*, International Institute of Scientific Travel Research, Geneva, 1953.

Lundberg : *International Travel and Tourism,* Institute of Certified Travel Agents, New York, 1970.

MacGregor, E. A. and C.T. Greenwood : *Polymers in Nature,* John Wiley & Sons, New York,

Mackinney, G. and A.C. Little : *Colour of Foods,* The AVI Publishing Company, Connecticut, 1972.

Malhotra, R. K. : *Fundamentals of Hotel Management and Operation,* Anmol Publications New Delhi, 1997.

Marton, I.D. and A.J.Macbod : *Food Flavours,* Elesvier Scientific Publishing Co., New York, 1982.

Mate, S. A. : *Cereal Sciences,* The AVI Publishing Co., Connecticut, 1969.

McIntosh, R.W. : *Hotel Principles, Practices and Philosophies,* Grid, Ohio, 1977.

Medlik, S. : *Higher Education and Research in Hotel Industry in Western Europe,* University of Surrey, London, 1966.

Mellor, J. D. : *Fundamentals of Freete-Drying,* Academic Press, London, 1978.

Michael Eskin, N.A. : *Plant Pigments, Flavours and Textures,* Academic Presss, New York, 1979.

Mill, R.C. : *The Hotel System,* Prentice-Hall International, London, 1985.

Morisson, A. M. : *Hospitality and Travel Marketing,* Delmar, New York, 1989.

Murthy, R.B. : *Breeding Procedures in Pearl Millet,* ICAR, New Delhi, 1977.

Nicholson, M. : *The Environmental Revolution,* Penguin, London, 1972.

Palmer, T. : *Understanding Enzymes,* John Wiley & Sons, New York, 1981.

Patmore, J. A. : *Land and Leisure,* David and Charles, London, 1970.

Pearce, D. : *Hotel Industry Organizations,* Longman, Harlow, 1992.

Pearce, Sales, J. : *Hotel Industry and Management Encyclopedia*, Blandford, London, 1959.

Peterson, M.S. and D.K. Tressler : *Food Technology the World Over*, The AVI Publishing Co., Connecticut, 1963.

Potter, N.M. : *Food Science*,The AVI Publishing Co., Connecticut, 1978.

Puruthi, J.S. : *Spices and Condiments*, National Book Trust of India, New Delhi, 1976.

Ranganna, K.S. and K.T. Achaya : *Indian Dairy Products*, Asia Publishing House, Bangalore, 1974.

Rao, D. V. : *Community and School Nutrition Education*, Discovery Publishing House, New Delhi, 1998.

Reilly, R. T. : *Hotel Management and Hotel Marketing Techniques*, Delmar, New York, 1988.

Rogers, C.A.C. : *Profitable Poultry Keeping in India and the East*, Treasure House of Books, Bombay, 1966.

Rudolph, Ballentine : *Diet and Nutrition*, The Himalayan International Institution, Honesdale, Pennsylvania, USA, 1979.

Runeckles, V.C. : *Recent Advances in Phytochemistry*, Academic Press, New York, 1972.

Ryan, C. : *Recreational Tourism : A Social Science Perspective*, Routledge, London, 1991.

Schultz, G.E. and R.H. Schirmer : *Principles of Protein Structure*, Springer-Verlage, New York, 1979.

Sheela, A. M. : *Economics of Hotel Management*, New Age Publishers, New Delhi, 1998.

Simms, A.E. : *History of Hotel Industry* , Virtue and Company Limited, London, 1973.

Smartt, J. : *Tropical Pulses*, Longman Group Ltd., London, 1976.

Stumbo,C.R. : *Thermobacteriology in Food Processing*, Academic Press, New York, 1998.

Swern, D, : *Bailey's Industrial Oil and Fat Products*, Interscience Publishers Division, John Wiley & Sons, New York, 1964.

Thankamma, J. : *Food Adulteration*, S.G. Wasani, New Delhi, 1976.

Turner, Louis and Ash John : *The Golden Hordes-International Tourism and the Pleasure Periphery*, Constable and Company, London, 1975.

Underwood, E.J : *Trace Elements in Human and Animal Nutrition*, Academic Press, New York, 1977.

Whistler, R.L. and J.N. BeMiller : *Industrial Gums*, Academic Press, New York, 1972.

Whiteley, P.P. : *Biscuit Manufacture*, Elsevier Publishing Co. Ltd., London, 1971.

Williams, J., R. E. Eakin, E. Beersteeker, and W. Shine : *The Biochemistry of Vitamins*, Reinhold, New York, 1950.

Yadav, C. P. : *Management of Hotel and Catering Industry*, Anmol Publications, New Delhi, 1998.

Index

H

I

J

K

L

M

N

O

P

❑❑❑